PRAISE FOR
Eat to Defeat Menopause

"Great recipes for menopausal women. Dr. Seibel and Ms. Giblin give us excellent food choices that will optimize our health during our most productive years. And the food is delicious!"

— Julia Johnson, MD, Chair, Department of Obstetrics & Gynecology, University of Massachusetts Medical School

"This is far more than a cookbook. It's practical advice and essential information on menopause. And if you follow the recipes . . . you will be happy, healthy, and helping the non-menopausal members in the family as well."

— Mary Jane Minkin, MD, Clinical Professor of Obstetrics & Gynecology and Reproductive Sciences, Yale University School of Medicine

eat to defeat
menopause

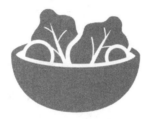

THE ESSENTIAL NUTRITION GUIDE FOR A HEALTHY MIDLIFE—WITH MORE THAN 130 RECIPES

A Red Hot Mamas® / HealthRock® Book

Karen Giblin & Mache Seibel, MD

Da Capo

LIFE
LONG

A Member of the Perseus Books Group

We would like to dedicate this book to our mothers,
who taught us the importance of a healthy diet and made us realize that the main difference
between an Italian mother and a Jewish mother is how they make the sauce, and to our children
who have been taught to "eat this, it's good, and it's good for you!"

Interior design by Pauline Brown

Set in 11 point Warnock Pro Light by the Perseus Books Group

Library of Congress Cataloging-in-Publication Data

Giblin, Karen L.
    Eat to defeat menopause : the essential nutrition guide for a healthy midlife—with more than 130 recipes / Karen Giblin & Mache Seibel.
        p. cm.
    Includes bibliographical references and index.
    ISBN 978-0-7382-1509-9 (pbk.)—
    ISBN 978-0-7382-1510-5 (e-book)
    1. Menopause—Diet therapy—Recipes. I. Seibel, Machelle M. II. Title.
RG186.G53   2011
618.1'750654—dc22   2011006062

First Da Capo Press edition 2011

Published by Da Capo Press
A Member of the Perseus Books Group
www.dacapopress.com

Da Capo Press books are available at special discounts for bulk purchases in the U.S. by corporations, institutions, and other organizations. For more information, please contact the Special Markets Department at the Perseus Books Group, 2300 Chestnut Street, Suite 200, Philadelphia, PA, 19103, or call (800) 810-4145, ext. 5000, or e-mail special.markets@perseusbooks.com.

10 9 8 7 6 5 4 3 2 1

CONTENTS

THE RECIPES

10   Pastas   119

11   Entrées   135

12   **Desserts**   191

FOREWORD

Many people tend to think of breakthroughs in medicine as a new drug, laser, or high-tech surgical procedure. They often have a hard time believing that the simple choices we make in our lifestyle—what we eat, how we respond to stress, whether or not we smoke, how much exercise we get, and the quality of our relationships and social support—can be as powerful as drugs and surgery, but they often are. Often, even better.

For more than thirty years, I have directed a series of studies showing what a powerful difference changes in diet and lifestyle can make. My colleagues and I at the nonprofit Preventive Medicine Research Institute showed, for the first time, that many diseases, including heart disease, prostate cancer, diabetes, and hypertension, are often reversible, and thus largely preventable.

We used high-tech, state-of-the-art measures to prove the power of simple, low-tech, and low-cost interventions.

We showed that integrative medicine approaches may stop or even reverse the progression of coronary heart disease, diabetes, hypertension, obesity, hypercholesterolemia, and other chronic conditions. We also published the first randomized controlled trial showing that these lifestyle changes may slow, stop, or even reverse the progression of prostate cancer, and may affect breast cancer as well.

Our latest research shows that changing lifestyle changes our genes in only three months—turning on hundreds of genes that prevent disease and turning off genes and oncogenes associated with breast cancer and prostate cancer, as well as genes that cause heart disease, oxidative stress, and inflammation. We also found that these lifestyle changes increase telomerase, the enzyme that lengthens telomeres, the ends of our chromosomes that control how long we live. Even drugs have not been shown to do this.

Although it's understandable that many people feel more bewildered than ever when they hear seemingly contra-dictory advice about different diets, there is actually a convergence of recommendations that is evolving. Some significant differences remain, but there is an emerging consensus among nutrition experts about what constitutes a healthy way of eating and living. It looks a lot like what you find in this book.

What you *include* in your diet is as important as what you *exclude.* There are at least 100,000 substances in foods that have powerful anticancer, anti–heart disease, and antiaging properties. These include phytochemicals, bioflavonoids, carotenoids, retinols, isoflavones, genistein, lycopene, polyphenols, and so on. Where do you find these potent substances? With few exceptions, these protective factors are found in fruits, vegetables, whole grains, legumes, soy products, and some fish. These are rich in good carbs, good fats, good proteins, and other protective substances. The recipes in this book are high in these protective substances.

You have a spectrum of choices. In all of our studies, we found that the more you change your lifestyle, and the more things you change, the better you feel and the healthier you become. And the better you feel, the easier it is to maintain these changes. Sustainable changes are based on joy, pleasure, and freedom, not deprivation and austerity.

It's not just about preventing illness or living *longer;* it's about living *better.* These lifestyle changes are likely to make you feel so much better, so quickly, that it reframes the reason for changing from fear of dying to joy of living.

When you eat and live healthier, your brain gets more blood so you think more clearly, have more energy, and need less sleep. You can even grow so many new brain cells that your brain can get measurably bigger in just a few months! Your skin gets more blood so you wrinkle less and look younger. Your sexual organs get more blood flow in the same way that drugs like Viagra work, so you enhance sexual potency. Now, *Eat to Defeat Menopause* describes how these same lifestyle changes can help empower and address the needs of menopausal women.

Dr. Seibel is a national expert in menopause and director of the Complicated Menopause Program at the University of Massachusetts Medical School, where he is also a professor. That, along with his books on soy, *The Soy Solution for Menopause,* and yoga, *A Woman's Book of Yoga,* provide him the wisdom and experience to offer readers much-needed information. Karen Giblin founded Red Hot Mamas Menopause Education Programs in 1991. These programs are held in hospitals within the United States and Canada. She has conducted numerous research projects and is nationally recognized for her work in women's health. They have combined health information and recipes to help women on their journey through menopause. The selections in this cookbook are from the authors and from chefs across the United States. The information on menopause and recipes in this book should be of great help to women as they search for easy-to-understand information about this sacred and transformative stage of life. I hope you find it to be useful.

Dean Ornish, MD
Founder and President, Preventive
Medicine Research Institute
Clinical Professor of Medicine,
University of California, San Francisco
Author, *The Spectrum*

ACKNOWLEDGMENTS

Just as many wonderful flavors and ingredients contribute to a great recipe, many wonderful people contributed to this cookbook. First, we would like to thank our spouses, Drs. Hjalmar Lagast and Sharon Seibel, for their encouragement and assistance, and for allowing us to spend hours of family time to work on this project. We also want to thank the many chefs and contributors who provided healthy, delicious recipes to help women *Eat to Defeat Menopause.*

Rachel Giblin and Cynthia Niles worked tirelessly to coordinate this book and bring it together. Thank you to our executive editor at Da Capo Press, Renée Sedliar, for her helpful insights in producing this high-quality book in a timely way, and to our agent, Kirsten Neuhaus, who identified a terrific publisher. We would like to offer a special thanks to Barbara Olendzki, RD, MPH, the nutrition program director of the Preventive and Behavior Medicine Department of the University of Massachusetts Medical School, and her associate Vijayalakshmi Patil, MS, RD, who ensured that the recipes were not only delicious but also calorie and fat conscious and in compliance with the Department of Health and Human Services recommendations.

Thanks to Darren Wheeling of Black Egg Syndicate for his beautiful illustrations, and to Karen Bressler, CEO of Agar Foods, who helped identify a number of the chefs who contributed. We also want to thank Dan Zaccagnini for his introduction to former White House chef Will Greenwood, and Allison Gallaher for her administrative efforts. In addition, we want to thank Dr. Dean Ornish, not only for providing the foreword to our book, but also for being an inspiration and teacher of healthy eating to us all.

Because we realize that not everyone in America has the opportunity to have nutritious meals every day, we are donating a portion of the proceeds from our book to three charities: Meals on Wheels, the Greater Boston Food Bank, and Community Servings of Boston.

INTRODUCTION

No illness which can be treated by diet should be treated by any other means.

—Moses Maimonides, AD 1200

This cookbook is for the Red Hot Mamas of the world. Yes, you! There are approximately 50 million of you in the United States alone. You are in or near menopause and you want to live long and be strong. And the best way to do that is to make wiser food choices, exercise, and watch your weight. That's important, since nearly one-third of adults are obese and have a body mass index (BMI) of 30 or greater. Menopausal women need between 1,800 and 2,200 calories per day, depending on their level of activity (see page 11). We want you to get the most from your calories by eating delicious and nutritious food so you eat healthy and don't gain weight. There are special nutritional needs of women in their menopausal years. Some of the phys-ical changes that occur are oftentimes inevitable. However, some of these changes may be due to bad habits that may not only make menopausal symptoms worse, but may also rob women of good health at menopause and beyond. And for the *mamas* and *bubbies* who enjoy cooking, our recipes are good for the whole family and are designed to introduce you to the world of delicious, healthy eating.

Eating well and exercising take some time and effort, and many women are at a loss as to where to begin. Our book offers a variety of suggestions on how to confidently prepare healthy foods that may affect the symptoms of menopause as well as different aspects of health. In essence, we show you how to eat healthy so you can stay healthy.

WHO ARE KAREN AND MACHE?

This is a special hello and welcome from the ethnic kitchens of two people whose day jobs are dealing with menopausal health and education. Karen's kitchen is Italian American and Mache's is Jewish American—and they both offer surprises and great recipes that *la famiglia* (Italian for "family") and *mishpokhe* (Yiddish for "family") alike will enjoy.

KAREN'S STORY

I grew up in an Italian American family, and that meant lots of love and lots of food and lots of food to love. My family actually brought over the first pizza recipe to Baltimore. They owned an Italian bakery and a well-known restaurant in a section of Baltimore called Little Italy. The restaurant was called DeNitti's. Of course, I was always told, "Eat this, it's good, and it's good for you!" I love to cook. And, yes indeed, to eat. Twenty years ago, I had a surgical menopause; I later founded the Red Hot Mamas, the largest menopause management education organization in this country and Canada, which provides women information—to arm them with knowledge—about the changes associated with the menopausal years. My Web site, www.redhotmamas.org, provides medically sound and valuable information to women across the world. I now want to go a step further and share some of my family recipes that provide better health and may lower the symptoms of menopause. I know for a fact that you can eat Italian meals, including a wonderful bowl of pasta, and enjoy every bite. However, you cannot eat pasta in unlimited amounts. In Italy, menopausal women are not fat, they're just super hot. And by hot, I mean that they have fabulous bodies at all ages. And forget the food adage that says, "Food that's good for you can't taste good." It's a myth. Our recipes prove that you can actually eat food that tastes good, *and* it will be good for you and your family.

MACHE'S STORY

I grew up in a Jewish American family where there was great food and continuous music. I spent some of my favorite time in Bubbie's kitchen as assistant chef and chief taster for recipes now known as "bubbielicious." The house became a magnet for family and friends because there was always good company, inviting music, and delicious food waiting. I was always told, "Eat this, it's good, and it's good for you!" As Bubbie entered menopause (shhhh . . . she's not talking age), she found even healthier ways to keep the same great taste. I learned to translate "a handful of this" and "a pinch of that" into fabulous recipes that are both healthy and nutritious. I also went to medical school, trained at Harvard, and became an expert in menopause, soy, and women's health. I founded HealthRock® to use music and songs to make health education fun and memorable—like Schoolhouse Rock, but for health. My Web sites have songs on health, wellness, and nutrition that are useful for menopausal women (and some of them are referenced in this cookbook). You can find *Recipe for Relaxation: Music for Body and Soul* and the Red Hot Mama CDs at www.healthrockwomen.com. It's music to chill and relax with while you cook and eat to defeat menopause. Now I want to share my healthy, delicious recipes and tell you why they're good for you.

HOW TO USE THIS COOKBOOK

Eat to Defeat Menopause is a little different from most cookbooks. This first section you're about to read has information about menopause. It also has some Red Hot Tips we think will be particularly helpful. We've provided useful tables and charts, "factoids" and "fictionoids," and foods to say yes to or to say no to, among other things. And, we may be the only cookbook to recommend a song to emphasize a key health message. *Eat to De-*

feat Menopause won't tell you how to exercise, though it will help you exercise good judgment to make the best food choices. It will give you the basic health and nutrition information you need so you can live long and stay healthy and strong. In addition to some great recipes we will give you from our own kitchens, we've also asked chefs from some of America's favorite restaurants to share some of their healthiest, most delicious recipes, to offer you an even wider range of wonderful choices. This is not a hot-flash cookbook, though some of the recipes will help to reduce hot flashes. But the ideas and recipes are not a flash in the pan. It's not a soy book like *The Soy Solution for Menopause;*[1] *Eat to Defeat Menopause* is a cookbook of healthy and delicious recipes created for you Red Hot Mamas. Read the text to learn about menopause, healthy eating, and nutrition tips. Use the recipes to have delicious meals that will be heart healthy, help you watch your weight, and may even help you reduce hot flashes. You'll also impress your friends and family because you will not only be a Red Hot Mama—you'll be a Red Hot Chef as well! Take the pause out of menopause, enjoy life, and thank you for letting us introduce you to the world of healthy and delicious eating. Eat to defeat menopause!

A NOTE ABOUT THE NUTRITIONAL ANALYSIS

The nutritional analyses were prepared using the Nutrition Data System for Research (NDSR). When a choice is given, the analyses are based on the first listed ingredient or quantity. Optional ingredients are not included. Phytoestrogens are valued by the sum of "isoflavones or similar."

KEY TO ABBREVIATIONS

Cal.	Calories (Kilocalories)
GI	Glycemic Index
Prot.	Protein
Carb.	Carbohydrate
SFA	Saturated Fatty Acids
MUFA	Monounsaturated Fatty Acids
PUFA	Polyunsaturated Fatty Acids
Calc.	Calcium
Sod.	Sodium
Pot.	Potassium

1

A LITTLE ABOUT PERIMENOPAUSE
AND MENOPAUSE

I'm not having a hot flash.
I'm having a power surge.

—ATTRIBUTED TO ALICE LOTTO STAMM

Every four minutes another American woman enters menopause. The infamous M-word. The Change. But it's okay. It's not the end. It's a new beginning. Women live one-third of their lives after menopause; and those same women who gave the world reproductive choice and the feminist movement want to know how to stay healthy, strong, and active forever. For many women, menopause, and the stage of life it represents, is very positive. You can't get pregnant, so there's more sexual freedom. And if the kids ever get a job and move out of the house, there is often more time and money to enjoy life. Fifty-one percent of postmenopausal U.S. women surveyed in a North American Menopause Society (NAMS)–sponsored Gallup Poll reported being happiest and most fulfilled between ages fifty and sixty-five, compared with when they were in their twenties.[1] Menopause is a relief to some women, especially if they have a positive outlook and establish good health practices. Lots of women have difficulty with their menstrual periods and are bothered by heavy bleeding, cramping, and PMS. So when menopause arrives, there is a newfound freedom. A new segment of life opens and women become more perceptive about the measures they take in achieving good health and wiser about their decision-making. They welcome menopause and make it the happiest days of their lives.

UNDERSTANDING THE LINGO

The word *menopause* has nothing to do with getting old. *Menopause* comes from two Greek words—*pausis* (cessation) and the root *men* (month)—it just means you don't have periods anymore. That's usually because a woman's ovaries no longer make enough estrogen to have a menstrual cycle (*natural* or *spontaneous* menopause). But it can also happen either when a woman's ovaries are removed by surgery (*surgical* menopause), or destroyed by radiation treatments, chemotherapy, or some other drug (*induced* menopause). A woman has to wait a full year after her last period to be sure it's menopause and not just a very irregular period (unless her ovaries are removed—*oophorectomy*). *Postmenopause* refers to all the years after

To hear the song "Red Hot Mama," go to www.healthrockwomen.com/music.

menopause. Having a hysterectomy (an operation to remove the uterus) stops menstruation, but it does not cause menopause unless the ovaries are also removed.

A hysterectomy is the most common major surgery performed in women in the United States—more than 600,000 each year. Hysterectomy, with or without removing the ovaries, causes more frequent and severe symptoms than natural menopause does, and that can make it more difficult to function at home or at work. As many as 75 percent of perimenopausal women in the United States have hot flashes. Their frequency usually increases during perimenopause, reaching the highest occurrence in the first two years of postmenopause, and then declining over time. Hot flashes are normal occurrences that happen to women at menopause. However, it's important to discuss hot flashes with your doctor as they also may be caused by other medical conditions. Having both your ovaries removed (bilateral oophorectomy) at the time of a hysterectomy (removal of your uterus) usually causes menopause to come on more abruptly; the sudden loss of estrogen causes more hot flashes.[2]

Even though women are living longer than ever before, the age of natural menopause hasn't changed much over the past few centuries—51.4 years. But any time between ages forty and fifty-five is normal. It often happens around the same time as to one's mother or sister. *Premature* menopause means it occurs before age forty, and that happens to about 1 to 2 percent of women. *Perimenopause* means "around menopause" and refers to the months and years (up to ten or twelve of the latter) leading up to menopause plus one year after menopause.

Ode to Soy and Hot Flashes

Drenched with sweat
I wake again
'Cause I'm afraid of estrogen
Can't recall how long it's been
Since I could sleep the night.
Trying soy could do no harm
It stopped the heat, though
I'm still warm.
Now I feel my life is charmed
'Cause I can sleep the night.
Experts say, "It's not the same
As estrogen," they all complain.
But it sure helped turn down
the flame.
And I can sleep the night!
—Mache Seibel, MD[3]

A NATURAL BRIDGE CROSSED OVER BY MANY

Baby boomers, those of us born from 1946 to 1964, are reaching our fifties and beyond, big time—about six thousand per day in United States. The same people who wanted to change the world in the 1960s are themselves starting to change. Today, if a woman reaches fifty without getting heart disease or cancer, she can expect to live to be ninety-two. Sixty is the new fifty. Menopause is just the next phase in a long life, complete with its benefits and its challenges. Realizing that menopause is a natural and inevitable next phase of life is valuable. It allows a person to stop asking, "How do I stop aging?" and begin asking the question posed by a prominent yogi, Hari Kaur Khalsa: "How do I remain graceful throughout life's challenges?"[4]

WHAT ARE PERIMENOPAUSE AND MENOPAUSE?

Yesterday is already a dream
And tomorrow is only a vision.
But today, well lived,
Makes every yesterday a dream of happiness
And every tomorrow a vision of hope.
—Anonymous

Ann Louise Gittleman begins her book *Before the Change* by saying, "Peri-what?" She goes on to ask the very question most other forty-plus-year-old women ask as they enter perimenopause and approach menopause: "What on earth is happening to my body?" Suddenly an active woman who is used to juggling her work while managing the household, carpooling the kids, and organizing the social calendar starts waking up at four AM with heart palpitations and feeling anxious and depressed. After a while she becomes a little more exhausted, a little more irritable, and notices she has a shorter attention span and a shorter fuse. Throw in a few mood swings, headaches, and trouble remembering where the car is parked, and suddenly you've got a woman convinced she is having a heart attack or has a brain tumor or a psychiatric problem. Sound familiar?

Many of the perimenopausal women we talk with have been to a doctor, had a normal EKG, and then are prescribed an antidepressant or a sleeping tablet for what seems like anxiety, depression, or a sleep disturbance. Many times the women don't realize that the root of their symptoms is, you guessed it, perimenopause.

HORMONES IN PERIMENOPAUSE AND MENOPAUSE

Ever ride a roller coaster? Ups and downs, right? That's what your hormones are like during menopause. Estrogen and progesterone levels plunge and soar and stop working together with precision. Your hormones act as though you're going through puberty, only backward. Remember how that felt? Wacky menstrual periods—often lighter but sometimes heavier, sometimes further apart, or even skipped, but often closer together. And when all of those mood swings and other symptoms kick in, it can feel like a raging case of PMS. And in many ways it is.

Like puberty, different women have different experiences. And why not? People are different before perimenopause, why shouldn't they be different during it? Fortunately, most women don't experience all of the symptoms of perimenopause. And the good news is, even though it is a challenge, perimenopause is only temporary.

- Hot flashes
- Insomnia
- Menses irregularities
- Memory problems (usually caused by disturbed sleep)
- Weight gain
- Vaginal dryness
- Heart palpitations
- Lower sexual desire
- Depression
- Anxiety
- Mood swings
- Bone loss

THERE IS MORE THAN ONE ESTROGEN

Your body makes three major estrogens. These are the ones everyone now calls *bioidentical* estrogens. Their names are estr*one* (E1), estra*diol* (E2), and estr*iol* (E3). Most of the estradiol is made in the ovaries. Some estrone is made in the ovaries, but it is mostly made in the body's fat cells. If you guess that women with more body fat make more estrone, you're right. More estrone is good news for some women because it may lower their symptoms of menopause. But women who are 25 to 50 pounds overweight have

a three-times-higher risk of uterine cancer, and if they are more than 50 pounds overweight, they are nine times as likely to get uterine cancer. On the other hand, women who are too thin and who have too little fat on their body may stop having periods because their body does not produce enough estrogen. These are the very reasons it's important to control your weight and that we want you to eat healthy!

ANALYSIS OF A HOT FLASH

What actually happens during a hot flash? The heat turns up, your heart speeds up, blood flow to the skin increases, and your face turns red. You are an official Red Hot Mama! Sweating often follows, particularly on the upper body. When the sweat evaporates a few minutes later, the body cools down and you may feel chilled.

Nobody knows for sure why hot flashes start. The thermostat that regulates your temperature is out of whack. Some tips to avoid them follow.

Will hot flashes happen to you? Most women will have at least some. Women who are too thin and who have lower blood estrogen levels are more likely to have hot flashes. And the lower the estrogen level, the more severe the hot flashes. The good news is that for most women, after three to five years, they begin to taper off.

Red Hot Tips to Help Avoid Hot Flashes:

- Avoid personal triggers. Everybody has them and you'll know yours. Examples are a warm room or using a hair dryer, psychological stress, or a confining space.
- Exercise regularly. It reduces stress and helps with sleep. Yoga, meditation, tai chi, or massage is particularly useful.
- Stay cool. Dress in light nightclothes, layer your bedding so you can take it off easily at night, keep a frozen cold pack under the pillow and turn your pillow often so the surface feels cool.
- Breathe deep and slow. When a hot flash begins, take slow, deep breaths through your nose and release out through your mouth. This is a great yoga technique.

2

WHAT DOES "HEALTHY WEIGHT" REALLY MEAN?

*There is no sincerer love
than the love of food.*

—GEORGE BERNARD SHAW

WOMEN AND WEIGHT GAIN

Weight gain is, well, a huge topic, especially in perimenopause and menopause. Hormonal changes may suddenly cause a woman's once curvy hourglass or pear-shaped figure to become more apple-shaped; it happens in part because lower estrogen levels can trigger fat to shift to the center of the body and accumulate around the belly. We've heard women describe this as "swelly bellies." A larger waist increases your chances of getting diabetes, high blood pressure, and heart disease.

Are you at increased risk? Measure your waist just above your belly button. A healthy waist measurement is less than 35 inches for a woman (less than 40 inches for a man), assuming your body mass index (BMI, see page 9) is less than 25.

CHANGES IN METABOLISM ARE THE NORM

Ever notice you can't eat as much as you used to without gaining weight?

Metabolism first starts to slow down during your thirties, causing the percentage of lean muscle in your body to decrease while fat increases. During your forties, things change even more. Your basal metabolic rate (BMR) drops by 4 to 5 percent each decade, making it even more important to eat healthy and to keep exercising. By the time you reach your fifties, your body needs 50 fewer calories each day than it did in your forties to not to gain weight. That is why it is so easy for pounds to sneak up on you if you waste your calories on poor food choices. Think healthy food choices! Think exercise! Think portion control!

In your sixties, most of any added weight will find its home in your abdominal area. Increasing girth increases your risk of high blood pressure, diabetes, and heart disease. By the seventh decade, it's common to lose muscle strength and tone and bone density. That's why we keep encouraging you to continue exercising, and if you can, to do weight training. And watch what and how much you eat. Burning off unwanted calories will help you fight off diseases and keep your muscles strong. It can also help keep your back straight so it doesn't hunch forward. See why this cookbook is making sense!

You know how they say as we get older we become more and more crea-tures of habit? It's true, even when it comes to food. A report in the *Journal of the American Medical Association* found that after a period of deliberate overfeeding, young men go back to eating less food, but elderly men continue to over-feed themselves. On the other hand, after a period of enforced underfeeding, young men increase their diet to make up for what they lost, but elderly men continue to underfeed themselves for up to ten days.[1] So if an older person has to stay in the hospital or gets depressed and starts to eat less, we can't assume that he or she will quickly start eating again once the problem passes. These types of situations can cause eating habits to change and have a major effect on a person's nutrition. It's important information, because between 30 and 50 percent of women sixty-five years and older are living alone, and are less likely to cook for themselves as well as more likely to either not eat or to go out and consume higher-caloric meals.

Other factors also play a role. About a third of people over age sixty make less acid in their stomach, a condition called *hypochlorhydria*. These changes make it harder to absorb vitamins B_6, B_{12}, and D, and riboflavin. In addition, our body makes vitamin D when our skin is exposed to sunshine. As we age, our skin changes and can't produce vitamin D as

TABLE 2.1 BODY MASS INDEX (BMI)

	21	22	23	24	25	26	27	28	29	30
5'0"	107	112	118	123	128	133	138	143	148	153
5'1"	111	116	122	127	132	137	143	148	153	158
5'2"	115	120	126	131	136	142	147	153	158	164
5'3"	118	124	130	135	141	146	152	158	163	169
5'4"	122	128	134	140	145	151	157	163	169	174
5'5"	126	132	138	144	150	156	162	168	174	180
5'6"	130	136	142	148	155	161	167	173	179	186
5'7"	134	140	146	153	159	166	172	178	185	191
5'8"	138	144	151	158	164	171	177	184	190	197
5'9"	142	149	155	162	169	176	182	189	196	203
5'10"	146	153	160	167	174	181	188	195	202	207
5'11"	150	157	165	172	179	186	193	200	208	215

well as it once did, so we need even more vitamin D. Since we need vitamin D to absorb calcium, less calcium gets absorbed, and that's bad for our bones. On top of this, nearly 75 percent of women of all ages don't consume enough calcium to keep their bones strong. Use this cookbook to help solve these problems. Low vitamin D levels also cause a loss of muscle strength and increase the risk of heart disease and breast cancer.

To hear the song "BMI," go to *www.healthrock women.com/music*. It's in the *Let's Move* CD.

AM I TOO FAT (OR TOO THIN)?

How do doctors determine if a person is under- or overweight? We use a tool called the body mass index (BMI). It's a formula[2] (weight in pounds ÷ height in inches × 703) that uses your weight and your height together. Look down the first column to find your height and then scan across to your weight. Your BMI is the number on top of that column. A BMI in the low 20s is the goal. Below 18.5 is underweight. A BMI of 25 to 29.9 is considered overweight and 30 or more is obese.

We can't blame all of this on hormonal changes. Two major culprits are poor eating habits and lack of exercise. The good news is you can rethink how you eat and eat to promote good health, shed some pounds, and focus on putting fitness back into your life.

DON'T WAIT TO LOSE WEIGHT

Losing weight is a simple concept—just eat fewer calories than your body uses. You can do that by eating healthy, controlling the size of your portions, exercising to burn more calories, or a combination of all three. Let this cookbook be your guide. This isn't a diet book. But if you stick with the recipes and information in this cookbook, you have a good chance of losing weight. And that's important. People in the United States and other industrialized countries are gaining 1 to 2 pounds per year. The IHRSA-sponsored study (Obesity/Weight Control Trend Report) conducted by American Sports Data, Inc., found that 3.8 million people in the United States weigh more than 300 pounds, 400,000 people (mostly men) weigh more than 400 pounds, and the average adult female weighs 163 pounds, which is 20 to 30 pounds overweight, depending on height. According to a report by the U.S. surgeon general, obesity causes 300,000 deaths every year. Some people are literally eating themselves to death!

The chart on page 11 shows the estimated amounts of calories (in kilocalories) needed to maintain energy balance for various gender and age groups at three different levels of physical activity. The estimates are rounded to the nearest 200 calories and were determined using the Institute of Medicine (IOM) equation.

EXERCISE

When Karen was young (she wasn't always a Red Hot Mama), her mother used to tell her, "When I was your age, I had to walk five miles to go to school." Her mom was encouraging her to become more active and be less dependent on being driven everywhere. Her mom also used to say, "You'll understand when you're older." Well, she was right. Exercise is as important as eating healthy. Look at the benefits of exercise:

- Reduces risk of heart disease and osteoporosis
- Controls weight
- Improves appearance and self-esteem
- Improves sleep
- Decreases depression by raising endorphins

TABLE 2.2 ESTIMATED DAILY CALORIE REQUIREMENTS (IN KILOCALORIES) FOR EACH GENDER AND AGE GROUP AT THREE LEVELS OF PHYSICAL ACTIVITY[a]

| Gender | Age (years) | Activity Level[b,c,d] | | |
		Sedentary[b]	Moderately Active[c]	Active[d]
Child	2–3	1,000	1,000–1,400[e]	1,000–1,400[e]
Female	4–8	1,200	1,400–1,600	1,400–1,800
	9–13	1,600	1,600–2,000	1,800–2,200
	14–18	1,800	2,000	2,400
	19–30	2,000	2,000–2,200	2,400
	31–50	1,800	2,000	2,200
	51+	1,600	1,800	2,000–2,200
Male	4–8	1,400	1,400–1,600	1,600–2,000
	9–13	1,800	1,800–2,200	2,000–2,600
	14–18	2,200	2,400–2,800	2,800–3,200
	19–30	2,400	2,600–2,800	3,000
	31–50	2,200	2,400–2,600	2,800–3,000
	51+	2,000	2,200–2,400	2,400–2,800

a These levels are based on Estimated Energy Requirements (EER) from the Institute of Medicine Dietary Reference Intakes macronutrients report, 2002, calculated by gender, age, and activity level for reference-sized individuals. "Reference size," as determined by IOM, is based on median height and weight for ages up to age 18 years and median height and weight for that height to give a BMI of 21.5 for adult females and 22.5 for adult males.

b *Sedentary* means a lifestyle that includes only the light physical activity associated with typical day-to-day life.

c *Moderately active* means a lifestyle that includes physical activity equivalent to walking about 1.5 to 3 miles per day at 3 to 4 miles per hour, in addition to the light physical activity associated with typical day-to-day life.

d *Active* means a lifestyle that includes physical activity equivalent to walking more than 3 miles per day at 3 to 4 miles per hour, in addition to the light physical activity associated with typical day-to-day life.

e The calorie ranges shown are to accommodate needs of different ages within the group. For children and adolescents, more calories are needed at older ages. For adults, fewer calories are needed at older ages.

When you exercise, try to get your heart to beat at 60 to 75 percent of its maximum capacity. This will give you the best cardiovascular benefit without over-taxing your heart. The desired heart rate changes with your age and your health. Try to exercise for an hour *at least* three times per week, with an emphasis on strength training, walking, and improving balance. This type of exercise helps to counter the loss in muscle mass that nat-urally occurs with aging as well as im-proving your metabolism, mood, and sleep. *Functional Fitness Starring Suzanne Andrews,* a show on PBS, offers excellent exercise routines to help you stay fit in the comfort of your own home (www .healthwiseexercise.com).

Always discuss with your doctor what is an ideal heart rate for you. An ad-visable range is listed below.

TABLE 2.3 TARGET HEART RATE

Age	Beats per Minute
20	120–160
25	117–156
30	114–152
35	111–148
40	108–144
45	105–140
50	102–136
55	99–132
60	96–128
65	93–124
70	90–120

Throughout this cookbook, we em-phasize fruits and vegetables, whole grains, lean meats, beans, and nuts. These foods will help you lose weight, especially if you substitute them for fats and starches, and limiting fat helps fight heart disease and some cancers. Eating more fruits and vegetables will also lower your chances of getting some types of cancer and other diseases such as diabetes. They also help to make sure your body gets the vitamins, minerals, and fiber it needs for good health.

The recipes in *Eat to Defeat Meno-pause* are calorie conscious and follow the dietary guidelines for Americans rec-ommended by the U.S. Department of Health and Human Services released in June 2010, so that the percent of calories per recipe is as follows:

Total Fat 30%

Saturated Fat 7–10%

Carbohydrates 50–55%

Protein 15–18%

To hear the song "Don't Be Afraid of a Squash," go to www.healthrockwomen.com/music. It's in the *Let's Move* CD.

Occasionally, one of the recipes might contain a little more fat or calories. We know everyone likes a special treat! You'll know by the number of calories so you can combine it with a salad or have fewer calories or fat in your next meal, so your eating experience for the day will stay healthy.

The average woman at menopause eats too many calories and consumes too much salt and sugar. Notice in the table on the previous page that after age thirty, women need fewer calories than when they were younger. The number of calories you need goes down even further after age fifty. This book offers information and recipes to improve health at menopause and beyond.

So, now let's separate fact from fiction about our diet and what may help us to lose weight.

DIET FACTOIDS AND FICTIONOIDS

There are a lot of misconceptions about our diet. Here are a few:

Fictionoid: *Skipping meals will help me lose weight.*

Factoid: Skipping meals can make us ravenously hungry. That makes us more likely to snack or eat more calories when we eat next. If you do need to snack, grab a piece of fruit or six to eight almonds or walnuts.

Fictionoid: *The best way to lose weight is to cut out starches (carbohydrates).*

Factoid: What we need to avoid are *simple* carbohydrates, such as refined sugar, concentrated sweeteners, honey, white flour, and alcohol. They are absorbed rapidly and make our body produce high levels of insulin that quickly lowers our blood sugar level, leaving us feeling hungry soon afterward. Insulin released like this also creates more fat on our body. On the other hand, *complex* carbohydrates, such as fruits and vegetables, whole grains, and legumes, are absorbed slowly so insulin levels don't have to quickly rise, and our blood sugar level stays more constant. White flour is whole wheat flour with the bran and fiber refined out of it. If you want pasta, just eat whole wheat pasta or whole wheat bread, or eat brown rice instead of refined rice, and voilà, you're eating complex carbohydrates.

Fictionoid: *I should cut out all fat from my diet.*

Factoid: The short answer is no, you shouldn't. You need at least 6 percent of the food you eat to be fat in order to make hormones and build cells, and for other important functions. But the average American diet is about 40 percent fat, and that increases your risk of heart disease.

The recommended amount of fat by most U.S. government agencies is 30 percent. According to Dr. Dean Ornish, from a weight-gain point of view, fat is fat whether it comes from healthy oils such as olive oil or from ice cream—a tablespoon of any fat, including olive oil, has 14 grams of fat, which is about the same as a scoop of ice cream. So if you eat a lot of fat from either oil or ice cream, you will gain weight.[3] From a health point of view, we should avoid *hydrogenated* or *trans fats* because they increase our risk of heart disease. Read the labels and limit these. Harvard researchers have shown that women who eat high levels of trans–fatty acids have a 50 percent greater risk of heart disease than those who eat the least.[4] "Good" fats are called *monounsaturated* fats (found in olive oil, canola oil, olives, some nuts, and avocados) or *polyunsaturated* fats (found in fish, seafood, soybeans, and whole grains).

Fictionoid: *The only way to lose weight is to starve yourself.*

Factoid: Not so. It is important to eat smart. A diet of largely complex carbohydrates that includes fruits, vegetables, whole grains, and legumes with moderate amounts of nonfat dairy and egg whites will fill you up—and help you lose weight. If you exercise and burn extra calories, all the better. Stay away from breads, use portion control, and don't keep eating once you feel full.

SOME RED HOT DIET TIPS

#1. AVOID LIQUID CANDY

What happens to your weight when you eat too much candy? It goes up, right? That's because candy has a lot of sugar and almost no nutrients that your body needs to stay healthy and strong.

We call soda "liquid candy," and here is why. There are 12 to 15 heaping teaspoons of sugar in every 12-ounce can of soda. In the 1950s, Americans drank four times as much milk as soda. Today, the U.S. Department of Agriculture says Americans drink almost four times as much soda as milk. How does this affect you?

To hear the song "Liquid Candy," go to www.healthrockwomen.com/music. It's in the *Let's Move* CD.

In 2004, doctors studied 51,603 women.[5] First, they made sure everything was the same except how much soda people drank. Here is what they found. Women who increased the number of sugar-sweetened carbonated soft drinks from one or fewer sodas per week to one or more sodas per day gained a lot of weight. Those women who went from one or more sodas per day to one or fewer sodas per week lost a lot of weight. And those women who did not change the amount of soda they drank did not have a change in their weight. They found the same thing was true for sweetened fruit punch.

You might think that just drinking a diet soda would solve the problem. Maybe not. Another report[6] studied what happened when men and women were give sugar-sweetened soda, artificially sweetened soda, or no soda for three weeks. Both men and women gained a lot of weight if they drank the sugar-sweetened sodas. But only the men lost weight if they drank the artificially sweetened soda. Here is the tip: Want an easy way to lose weight? Stop drinking soda and other sweetened drinks and drink more water and nonfat milk.

#2: UNDERSTANDING THE GLYCEMIC INDEX

Did you know that carbohydrates are not all created equal? Some, such as a soda or a potato, can quickly raise your blood sugar. Others, such as fruits and vegetables (besides potatoes), don't raise your blood sugar level much at all. How quickly a carbohydrate increases your blood sugar level is given a value called the glycemic index (GI).[7] Foods are ranked from 0 to 100. Pure glucose has a value of 100. Choosing carbohydrates with medium or low GI can help you lose weight, reduce the risk of heart disease, control diabetes, reduce hunger feelings, and keep you fuller longer.

How does this happen? When your blood sugar rises quickly, it triggers a large release of the hormone insulin to bring your blood sugar level back down to normal. That quick lowering of your blood sugar causes you to feel hungry again in a few hours. Did this ever happen to you? If you said yes, it's time to change that. Over time, a high-GI diet will increase your risk of diabetes, heart disease, and even cancer. Choosing carbohydrates with a medium or low GI keeps your blood sugar level more constant and lowers your risk of those diseases and obesity.

That's why the recipes in this cookbook include their GI. You can find out more about GI at www.glycemicindex.com.

Low GI = 55 or less

Most fruits, vegetables (except potatoes and watermelon), grainy breads, milk, soy milk and other soy products, fish, eggs, meat, beans and peas, nuts, and brown rice have a low GI.

Medium GI = 56 to 69

Whole wheat products, basmati rice, and sweet potatoes have a medium GI.

High GI = 70 or more

Many breakfast cereals, baked potatoes, white bread, instant white rice, and doughnuts have a high GI.

The glycemic load (GL) tells you how much of a carbohydrate is in a serving of a particular food. So if a food has a high GI, such as watermelon, but there isn't a lot of sugar in it, its GL is low. Here is a tip: If you choose to eat a high-GI food, eat a smaller portion so the GL stays medium to low. Here are the values to look for:

High GL = 20 or more
Medium GL = 11 to 19
Low GL = 10 or less

3

DIETARY STRATEGIES FOR HOT FLASHES, INSOMNIA, AND OTHER MENOPAUSAL SYMPTOMS

Let your food be your medicine,
and your medicine be your food.

—HIPPOCRATES

Hippocrates said it best. This chapter outlines some of the most common symptoms of menopause, along with tasty, nutritional suggestions that may reduce or eliminate them.

HOT FLASHES AND INSOMNIA

One of the reasons we wrote this book is that what you eat and drink can affect menopausal symptoms. We want all of you Red Hot Mamas to eat to defeat menopause. Here are some Red Hot Tips that may reduce hot flashes and help with sleep:

SAY YES TO:

Foods that contain phytoestrogens, which may help reduce hot flashes. These include soy foods such as edamame and soy nuts, tofu, and soy yogurt or milk. Also, flaxseeds, sesame seeds, garlic, hummus, and veggie burgers are a few items that provide phytoestrogens.

Carbohydrates and other sleep-promoting foods. Carbohydrate-rich foods may help if you are losing your snoozing time due to sleep issues. Studies suggest that eating carbs can increase the release of tryptophan, an amino acid that helps the brain manufacture the chemical serotonin, which helps people fall asleep. Try eating a piece of toasted whole-grain bread, or a small portion of another carbohydrate, before going to bed. Other foods that contain tryptophan are turkey, soy, cod, egg whites, and warm milk. Tryptophan helps promote sleep. Also, omega-3 fatty acids, which are found in fish such as salmon, trout, and tuna, play a role in sleep induction. And don't forget cherries. They contain melatonin, a substance found in the body, which helps regulate sleep.

SAY NO TO:

Large meals. When you eat a large meal, the body's digestion brings blood into the abdomen, raises body temperature, and voilà, tells the hypothalamus part of the brain to send a signal that causes hot flashes. Eating smaller meals can help reduce the number of hot flashes.

Caffeine. Coffee, tea, colas, and even dark chocolate contain caffeine. They may trigger hot flashes as well as affect the quality of your sleep. So drink more water and avoid caffeine, especially in the late afternoon and at night. Substitute decaffeinated beverages, teas that are caffeine free, and water. Too much caffeine can also take calcium out of your bones.

Alcohol. Alcohol can increase the number and intensity of hot flashes and affect sleep, mood swings, and your weight. Heavy alcohol use can even lead to osteoporosis because it prevents bone cells from building new bone. Too much alcohol also increases the chances of falling and breaking a bone. And there may be an even more important reason to limit alcohol: We've been told for a decade that drinking a glass of red wine every day may be good for your heart. But several recent studies have found that drinking as little as one alcoholic beverage a day can increase a woman's chances of getting breast cancer. Play it safe—limit yourself to no more than one drink a day. Here is another Red Hot Tip: If you are going to a cocktail party, always eat something solid *before* you get there, so you won't go overboard on the appetizers.

Hot, spicy foods. Cayenne, chile peppers, wasabi, and hot mustard can turn up the heat.

HEADACHES

Headaches are a common problem during the menopause transition. They seem to increase at perimenopause, and hormone fluctuations may play a role in causing them. They also may be due to changes in our sleeping patterns. Daily supplementation with magnesium, vitamin B$_2$ (riboflavin), and/or coenzyme Q10 is an effective and safe option for women who experience headaches.

SAY YES TO:

Foods that are rich in magnesium, such as almonds, black beans, broccoli (raw), halibut, okra, oysters, and scallops, among others.

SAY NO TO:

Alcohol (especially red wine), *foods that contain monosodium glutamate (MSG), and cured meats* such as salami and bologna.

BLOATING

During the menopause transition, another common midlife symptom is bloating, which may be due to hormone fluctuations, an overproduction of estradiol, and the conversion of androgen (a so-called "male" hormone) to estrogen through a process called *aromatization,* which increases with age and body weight.

SAY YES TO:

Foods and herbs that have diuretic properties, such as celery seeds, parsley, dandelion, juniper berries, asparagus, artichokes, melon, and watercress. And drink plenty of water and herbal teas.

SAY NO TO:

Sugary and high-sodium foods such as frozen dinners and canned soups. Read the sugar and sodium content on food labels, and reduce the amount of sugar and salt you add to foods and beverages.

MOOD SWINGS

Many women during the menopause transition report symptoms of a decreased sense of well-being due to mood disturbances such as irritability and mood swings. Your food choices may be linked to some of these mood changes. When women eat better, they feel better. Good nutrition plays a major role in our moods. So it is important to understand which foods stabilize our moods and which ones to avoid.

SAY YES TO:

Omega-3 fatty acids foods such as tuna, salmon, and mackerel. Eat vegetables such as asparagus, Brussels sprouts, and beets, which are rich in B vitamins. Green vegetables such as spinach and peas are high in folic acid, a member of the B-complex group that may also help stabilize your mood because it's needed to make serotonin. Always use fresh vegetables whenever you can and don't forget that spinach and other dark, leafy greens can be used raw in salads and sandwiches as well. Chicken and turkey are also rich in vitamin B, which may also play a role in the production of serotonin in the body.

SAY NO TO:

Sugary foods, which cause a rise in your blood sugar and may increase mood disturbances.

DECREASED SEX DRIVE

For some women, menopause and its associated decline in "sex" hormones can lead to a decline in sex per se. Lower levels of estrogen is the main culprit and that can lower libido and cause vaginal dryness. If that happens to you, can food spice up your sex life? Recent information suggests that it can, though medical science is still scratching its head with skepticism. So let's take a look at some foods that *may* spice up your sex life.

SAY YES TO:

Granola, oatmeal, nuts, dairy, green vegetables, garlic, soybeans, and chickpeas. These foods contain L-arginine, which is thought to be helpful in improving sexual function.

Avocados contain potassium, which regulates thyroid hormones and may enhance female libido.

Chocolate intake releases serotonin in the brain, producing feelings of pleasure similar to having sex. Chocolate also contains phenylalanine, which raises endorphins, making us feel good and less depressed. But sisters, indulge in moderation for its benefit, and try eating it as a prelude to lovemaking.

Asparagus is a vegetable to consider due to its vitamin E content. At nineteenth-century weddings, asparagus was served because of its reputation as an aphrodisiac.

Fresh fruits. Feast on fresh fruits such as strawberries, pomegranates, and grapes, which are rich in antioxidants and are not only sensual but delicious.

Chile peppers. Eating chile peppers triggers the release of endorphins, those natural opioids that create a high that is like lovemaking. But remember, chile peppers can also trigger hot flashes.

SAY NO TO:

Alcohol, which affects blood flow and impacts testosterone levels and libido, contributing to sexual dysfunction. Alcohol can cause both women and men to experience a reduction in sexual arousal and difficulty having orgasms, and men may have difficulty getting an erection.

OSTEOPOROSIS (THINNING OF THE BONES)

If you are a Red Hot Mama, it's important that you bone up on how to prevent osteoporosis. Here is why: A healthy fifty-year-old woman is just as likely to die of a complication of osteoporosis as she is to die of breast cancer. You may already have had a mammogram. But have you gotten a bone density test? According to the National Osteoporosis Foundation, osteoporosis is a major health threat for an estimated 44 million Americans, or 55 percent of the people fifty years of age and older. Ten million individuals already have the disease and almost 34 million more are estimated to have low bone density, which increases their risk for osteoporosis and broken bones. Eighty percent of those affected by osteoporosis are women. Every twenty seconds, another American breaks

Red Hot Tips and Habits You Can Change to Keep Bones Strong:

- If you smoke—quit!
- Exercise 30 minutes three to five times a week. Jogging, jumping rope, walking briskly, or lifting weights can increase bone density 3 to 5 percent per year.
- Limit alcohol to one glass of wine, one beer, or 1 ounce of spirits daily.
- Avoid high caffeine use.
- Limit salt and sodas; they increase calcium loss through your kidneys.
- Get 1,200 mg of calcium, 400 to 800 IU of vitamin D, and 400 mg of magnesium daily. If you don't get that much in your diet, take supplements.
- Eat healthy. Some of the recipes in this book can help lower your risk of osteoporosis and keep your bones strong.
- Check your vitamin D blood level. So many Red Hot Mamas have low levels and it's easy to fix with supplements. You can't absorb calcium without enough vitamin D and it might help protect against breast cancer.

a bone because of osteoporosis. Nearly half of all women over fifty will break a bone because of osteoporosis. One in four men will, too. By 2025, experts predict osteoporosis will cost the country over $25 billion annually.[1]

To hear the song "Osteoporosis," go to www .healthrockwomen.com/music. It's in the *Women's Edition* CD.

But there is no need to tiptoe around, afraid that calcium is silently oozing out of your bones, leaving you frail and vulnerable. Get a bone density test as menopause approaches. They have only 10 percent of the radiation received in a routine chest X-ray, and they diagnose the problem.

4

UNDERSTANDING SOY FOODS
THE PERFECT FOOD FOR MENOPAUSE

He that takes medicine and neglects diet wastes the skills of the physician.

—CHINESE PROVERB

Soy is one of the healthiest foods you can eat. It has lots of protein, minerals, vitamins, and a whole lot more. Soy contains *phyto*estrogens, or "plant" estrogens—plant substances that mildly mimic weak estrogens in your body. There are so many ways to prepare it, so many ways to incorporate it into your daily diet, and so many ways to cook it, we're sure you can find a way to enjoy it. Especially when you realize that although the data is inconclusive, soy may help some women's hot flashes and might even have other health benefits.[1]

SOYBEANS AND FOODS MADE DIRECTLY FROM THEM

SOYBEANS

Soybeans come in several colors, depending on when they are harvested. The green ones that look like fuzzy Chinese snow peas are still slightly immature. They are called *edamame.* Later in the season, soybeans begin to dry and turn yellow, black, or brown. They look like black-eyed peas without the black eye.

Canned soybeans are ready to be used and can be added to chilis, stews, and soups right out of the can. Using the liquid in the can will save some of the B vitamins that might be lost from the canning process.

Dried soybeans, like most other legumes, have to be soaked overnight to rehydrate them. It usually takes about 3 cups of water for each cup of soybeans. In the morning, drain off the water, cover them again with fresh water, simmer over low heat for 3 hours, and they are ready to be used in recipes.

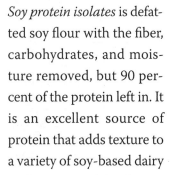

If you're using a tomato product in your recipe, it's better to add it when the dish is nearly done because tomatoes toughen the outer layer of the bean, making it take longer to soften. After soybeans are cooked, eat them within the next few days.

SOY FLOUR

Soy flour is made by grinding up whole, dried soybeans. It can't be used by itself, but it can replace up to 20 percent of the weight of all-purpose flour required in almost any recipe. You can also use soy flour as a substitute for eggs in recipes by adding 1 tablespoon of soy flour and 2 tablespoons of water for each egg called for.

SOY POWDER

Soy powder is very similar to soy flour. The difference is that the soybeans are cooked before they are ground. It can be used to make soy milk, added as powdered milk to coffee, or added to recipes in place of other ingredients.

SOY PROTEIN ISOLATES

Soy protein isolates is defatted soy flour with the fiber, carbohydrates, and moisture removed, but 90 percent of the protein left in. It is an excellent source of protein that adds texture to a variety of soy-based dairy foods, such as cheese, nondairy frozen desserts, and coffee whiteners. It's also a major ingredient in soy hot dogs, soy ice cream, baby food, and meat analogues.

TEXTURED VEGETABLE PROTEIN (TVP)

Textured vegetable protein is a modern Western invention. Defatted soy flour is compressed until its protein fiber changes in structure. When water is added to it, the TVP gets very coarse, so it looks and feels like ground beef. Add a little chicken or beef flavoring and you've got a stew or the perfect taco or chili meat substitute. Added (up to 20 percent or less by weight) to your next hamburger dish, it is the perfect hamburger extender; you can't taste the difference, but you will be getting 20 percent less animal fat from the same dish.

SOY GRITS

Soy grits come from the whole bean, so they taste a lot like soybeans and retain 55 to 65 percent of the protein by weight and most of soy's beneficial contents. They are made by lightly toasting and hulling the soybeans, then either cracking or grinding them into small pieces. Because soy grits contain most of the fat of the beans, they become rancid if not refrigerated. You can use soy grits as a breakfast cereal by stirring one part grits into three parts boiling water, then cover, lower the heat, and simmer until all the water is absorbed. It's not an instant breakfast, though. Unless the beans are presoaked, cooking takes about 45 minutes. Soy grits are a bit chewy, so they're a natural extender for hamburger or a great way to add texture to chili, stews, and spaghetti sauce.

SOY SPROUTS

Soy sprouts are an excellent source of magnesium, folic acid, and vitamin C, and they are low in sodium. You can add them fresh to salads or cook them fast at low heat.

SOY MILK AND PRODUCTS MADE FROM IT

SOY MILK

Soy milk is an ancient drink, developed by Chinese Buddhist monks who then brought it to Japan. Soy milk was first available in the United States in the 1920s. Asians drink it daily the way cow's milk is consumed in the West. Once the carton is opened, it must be refrigerated and used up within about a week. Soy milk can be used for anything you use milk for, such as on dry cereal and instead of milk to make cream of wheat or oatmeal. But you can also use it to make sauces, puddings, custards, or mousse (Note: For the latter three items, some kind of starch, such as arrowroot or agar, will need to be added to make the dairy-free items thicken). Soy milk is rich in iron, phosphorus, thiamine, copper, potassium, and magnesium, as well as vegetable protein.

OKARA

Okara is the pulp and hulls that remain after the soy milk is strained. Its name literally means "honorable hull." It is very high in fiber and protein. Okara is often described as having a coconut-like texture, which makes it a frequently used ingredient in granola bars, muffins, and cookies. It can also be found in vegetarian burgers. Keep your okara refrigerated and use it within a few days.

YUBA

Yuba is the "skin" that forms on soy milk when it is heated. It isn't usually available in the United States, but it can be found widely in China and in gourmet shops in Japan, where it is considered a delicacy. Yuba is 52.4 percent protein and is commonly added to soups and stews. It can also be pressed into molds and made into imitation meat.

SOY CHEESE

Soy milk can be made into cheeses just as cow's milk can. It is low in fat and cholesterol, and lactose free. If it is held together with calcium caseinate, that means it contains dairy. If isolated soy protein is used, it is dairy free. Like soy milk, it is available full fat, low fat or fat free as mozzarella, Jack, and Cheddar.

SOY YOGURT

Soy yogurt is a dairylike product made by adding live bacteria cultures to soy milk. A 1-cup serving contains 12 grams of soy protein, no lactose (check label to be sure), and no cholesterol. You can buy it plain or with fruit added, and as whole or low fat. Soy yogurt has a similar consistency to dairy yogurt so you can use it interchangeably for a snack or as an ingredient in foods such as sauces, milk shakes, and desserts.

TOFU

Tofu is also known as *bean curd* and *doufu*. It's inexpensive and easy to digest for young and old. After a curdling agent is added to soy milk, it separates into curds and whey. Tofu is the soybean curds that are compressed into the white, spongy cubes seen in most health food stores and supermarkets. It comes in several forms, all of which have to be kept refrigerated, except the dried variety. Keep any unused portion submerged in water and change the water daily. Tofu acts as a flavor sponge—it soaks up the flavor of whatever it is cooked with. Crumble a block of firm tofu in your hand and add it to hamburger and it tastes like hamburger. Cut it into cubes and add it to soup, or stir-fry it with your favorite seasonings and vegetables. The softer forms of tofu are sweeter and make a great choice for combining with your favorite fruits and whipping up in the blender. They also make great puddings and cream pies because they take up the taste of the chocolate or whatever flavor you add.

FERMENTED FORMS OF SOY

Fermented forms of soy are very common, particularly in Asian restaurants. They have many positive qualities but generally do contain high amounts of salt. Be sure to read the labels.

TEMPEH

Tempeh (pronounced TEM-pay) is made from whole soybeans cooked with a mold, *Rhizopus,* from the hibiscus plant, at a warm temperature for 18 to 24 hours. The tempeh emerges as a chunky bean cake covered with an edible white mold. Tempeh has a strong, distinctive taste with a chewy consistency that makes it a great meat substitute. You can marinade it and barbecue or grill it, steam it, or prepare it as you would tuna fish by grating it up and mixing it with mayonnaise, celery, and onions. A 3-ounce serving has about 150 calories, 16 grams of protein, and 6 grams of fiber. It you notice small gray or black flecks in your tempeh, it just means that it is naturally fermented. You can refrigerate it for up to a week or freeze it for up to several months.

NATTO

Natto is another fermented soy food made from cooked whole soybeans. It is made by mixing in a bacteria culture with the soybeans and allowing them to ferment in plastic bags. In Japan it is used as a spread, at breakfast or dinnertime, or with shoyu (traditional soy sauce) and mustard. Natto is high in protein and rich in fiber, but lower in sodium than either miso or soy sauce. It's also a good source of iron and other minerals, and B vitamins. If you are taking a class of antidepressants called MAO inhibitors, be careful eating natto. It contains the amino acid tyramine, which can dangerously elevate your blood pressure.

MISO

Miso is made with soybeans alone or soybeans combined with a grain, such as barley or rice, together with salt and a mold culture. Before being used, it is left for up to three years in a cedar vat to ferment. It comes in a smooth and a chunky variety. A tablespoon of miso has 680 milligrams of sodium compared with table salt, which has 6,589 milligrams of sodium. Miso is a great source of protein (12 to 21%), comparable to eggs (13%), or even chicken (20%). Like natto, it contains the amino acid tyramine that can increase your blood pressure if you are taking a class of antidepressants known as MAO inhibitors.

SOY SAUCE

Everyone who has gone out for Chinese food sees *soy sauce* either on the table or in the packet you come home with. The soy sauce we know in America is different from the traditional soy sauce in Asia that is known as *shoyu*. Shoyu is made by adding a mold to cooked soybeans and a grain, then fermenting them in salty brine for one to one and a half years. The soy sauces we're used to buying in bottles at the supermarket are really defatted soybean meal and wheat mixed with chemicals, corn syrup, and food coloring. Shoyu is sometimes called *tamari,* but that name is also used for the liquid that is left over when miso is made.

5

MORE HELPFUL FOODS FOR MENOPAUSE AND OTHER DIETARY GUIDELINES

There are other important foods besides soy that you ought to know about to optimize your journey as a Red Hot Mama. In addition, we'll discuss some important guidelines to help you understand better how to eat to defeat menopause.

FLAXSEED

Flaxseed is another food that has been eaten for thousands of years. Flaxseeds are still popular in Asia, Scandinavia, and Africa. They look a lot like sesame seeds, except they are dark brown and have a pleasant nutty taste. In ancient times they were known as linseed, and the plant's fibers were woven into cloth, paper, and rope. In fact, the Egyptians used this type of cloth for wrapping mummies. Flaxseeds contain about 18 percent protein and provide calcium, potassium, and B vitamins. They also contain boron, a micronutrient considered important in conditions such as arthritis and that may enhance levels of the body's own estrogen. In addition, flaxseeds are a rich source of the phyto-estrogens known as *lignans.* Many women say that flaxseed helps reduce their hot flashes, but there is still only a small amount of scientific data to support their reports. If you do want to use flaxseeds to help with hot flashes, try eating 1 to 2 tablespoons of flaxseed oil daily, grinding up flaxseeds and spreading them on your salad or adding them to your cereal, or consider adding to your diet some of Zoe Foods' new Flax & Soy cereals and bars. Flaxseeds are also high in soluble fiber. In fact, soaking them overnight in water turns the flaxseeds into a gelati-nous mass that makes a gen-tle fiber and a great cooking ingredient. You can also grind up the seeds to make flaxseed cereals, crusts, and snack bars. Flaxseeds can also be found as powders that are more a laxative than a cooking ingredient, and flax oil, which usually does not have many lignans because they stay behind with the residue of the seeds. Flax oil is a source of omega-3 fatty acids. Ground flaxseeds and water also make a great egg substitute in recipes. (For the equivalent of one egg, mix one 1 tablespoon of ground flaxseeds with 3 tablespoons of water; stir until com-bined.) Be sure to buy only fresh, refrig-erated flax oil in opaque bottles that have an expiration date. When it's fresh it has a nutty taste. When it's old it tastes bitter and even a bit like fish oil. When that hap-pens, throw it out and buy a new bottle.

OMEGA-3 FATTY ACIDS (FISH OIL)

Did your mother ever give you cod liver oil? Once again, Mother knew best! Fish oil contains a lot of omega-3 fatty acids. Studies show omega-3s are a type of fat that lowers your risk of heart disease and helps to lower cholesterol, and they are good for your joints and your brain. Omega-3s may even help your skin look good. How much do you need? Eating fish twice a week or taking a daily supple-ment containing 800 to 1,000 milligrams (0.8 to 1 gram) should be about right. Be-cause fish does contain mercury, which can be bad for you, if you want to eat more fish or take higher doses of supple-ments, talk with your doctor. Our cook-book has included a number of great recipes that contain fish and seafood as a delicious way to get your omega-3s. Here are some examples of how to get 1.5 grams of omega-3s by eating different types of fish:[1]

Anchovies, herring, mackerel,
  salmon: 1 serving (3 ounces)
Albacore tuna, sablefish, sardines:
  1¼ servings (3.75 ounces)
Bluefin tuna, trout: 1½ servings
  (4.5 ounces)
Halibut, swordfish: 2 servings
  (6 ounces)
Freshwater bass, oysters:
  2½ servings (7.5 ounces)
Sea bass: 3 servings (9 ounces)
Shrimp, pollack: 3½ servings
  (10.5 ounces)

EAT YOUR VEGGIES!

Do you remember Popeye holding a can of spinach? He knew that green leafy vegetables are good for you. Spinach has only 30 calories per cup and is a great source of calcium, potassium, and vitamins, and it helps protect us from diseases such as osteoporosis, heart disease, and colon cancer. A July 2009 article in the British journal *Cancer* found that vegetarians are 12 percent less likely to develop cancer than are meat eaters, and 45 percent less likely to develop certain cancers, such as cancers of the blood, stomach, and bladder.[2] That's because vegetables have antioxidants, substances that prevent pieces of molecules from connecting together to form cancer-causing chemicals.

In general, fresh spinach contains a lot more vitamins than the canned stuff Popeye ate. And you don't have to wait until dinner to have vegetables. You can put spinach or sautéed asparagus in an egg-white omelet or in a salad or sandwich, or you can add it to a pot of soup. One cup of cooked kale has more calcium than a cup of milk. Other calcium-rich vegetables include collard greens, chard, broccoli, and dandelion leaves, to name a few. Steaming is an excellent way to cook vegetables because it prevents loss of vitamins and minerals in cooking and it's fast and easy to do. Try to stay away from creamed vegetables. They may taste good, but the extra calories will lead to unwanted weight and the cream isn't heart healthy. Keep your refrigerator stocked with other vegetables that are healthy and crunchy and can be eaten raw. Instead of going for the M&M's, reach for radishes, carrots, cucumbers, broccoli, bell peppers, blanched green beans or snow peas, cherry tomatoes, or soy nuts, all of which will satisfy that craving for something crunchy many of us get, particularly before the dinner hour. Make a healthy salad with roasted vegetables, black olives, beans, and a healthy protein such as tuna or tofu. Choose a wide variety of salad greens, including arugula, spinach, watercress, and more. Don't be afraid of a squash!

OTHER DIETARY GUIDELINES

There is a lot of talk about cholesterol and sometimes it can be confusing. The government also has created dietary guidelines that have gone through some changes. We've tried to explain these important dietary facts to keep you on the path of being a Red Hot Mama.

UNDERSTANDING CHOLESTEROL

Cholesterol is a waxy, fatlike substance that is part of every cell in our body—our brain, nerves, muscles, skin, liver, intestines, and heart. Our body also uses cholesterol to make vitamin D and many hormones, including estrogen. But when our body has too much cholesterol, it can end up lining our blood vessels, making them narrower and hard and increasing our risk of heart disease. And heart disease is the number one cause of death for women in menopause. So the recipes in this cookbook focus on keeping your cholesterol levels down. In addition to cholesterol, there are several other kinds of fats in our blood. Because high blood cholesterol increases your risk of having a heart attack, it's important to check your cholesterol levels regularly and know what the results mean. Here is some general information to help you understand "the numbers."

WHAT DO MY CHOLESTEROL LEVELS MEAN?[3]

Total Blood Cholesterol

Desirable Level: Less than 200 mg/dL (milligrams per deciliter of blood)
Borderline High: 200 to 239 mg/dL
High Risk: 240 mg/dL and higher

HDL ("Good") Cholesterol

HDL stands for *high-density lipoprotein.* HDL is considered the "good" cholesterol because it protects you from having a heart attack. It's different from the other cholesterol levels—the higher your HDL, the better. Several things can help you increase your HDL level: Quit smoking, lose excess weight, eat a good diet (see why we're doing this cookbook?), and exercise. It's simple—healthy lifestyle changes can increase your HDL and decrease your risk of heart attack.

	For Men	*For Women*
Desirable HDL Level:	45 mg/dL *or higher*	55 mg/dL *or higher*
At Risk:	Less than 35 mg/dL	Less than 45 mg/dL

LDL ("Bad") Cholesterol

LDL stands for *low-density lipoprotein.* It's part fat and part protein. LDL is made in the liver and travels in the blood to the tissues of the body. A high level of LDL means there is a higher risk of heart disease. If you already have heart or vascular disease or diabetes, many doctors want your LDL level to be less than 100 mg/dL, or even less than 70 mg/dL.

> Desirable Level: Less than 130 mg/dL
> Borderline: 130 to 159 mg/dL
> High: 160 mg/dL or higher

What should my TRIGLYCERIDE level be?

Triglycerides are a type of lipid. The American Heart Association defines triglycerides as the chemical form in which most fat exists in food as well as in the body. They are called *triglycerides* because in their molecular form, they contain three molecules of fatty acids held together with glycerol. When you eat, your body converts any calories it doesn't need to use right away into triglycerides. The triglycerides are stored in your fat cells. Later, hormones release triglycerides for energy between meals. If you eat too many calories, you will get elevated triglycerides in your blood. Being overweight, drinking a lot of alcohol, and eating refined carbohydrates and saturated fats can increase your triglyceride level. Diabetes and some other medical problems can also increase your triglyceride level, which can put you at risk of coronary artery disease, low HDL levels, high blood pressure, and diabetes.

> Normal: Less than 150 mg/dL
> High: 150 to 400 mg/dL
> Very High: Greater than 400 mg/dL

> To watch the video *Trans Fats,* go to www.youtube.com/HealthRockTV.

UNDERSTANDING THE NEW FOOD PYRAMID[4]

Every five years, the Departments of Agriculture (USDA) and Health and Human Services (HHS) join forces to write new dietary guidelines. The most recent guide, *MyPyramid.gov: Steps to a Healthier New You,* was published in June 2010.

Here are the key points you need to know:

1. *Grains:* Wheat, rice, oats, cornmeal, barley, and other cereals are grains. Make half your grains whole and avoid refined grains because they remove the bran and germ portions of the grain kernel, which also removes the fiber. If you do eat refined grains, make sure they are *enriched,* meaning the makers put back

in the B vitamins and iron that are removed during the refining process. The fiber in whole grains helps you eat more slowly and fill up naturally, and this helps prevent overeating.

    a. Eat at least 3 ounces of whole-grain bread, cereal, crackers, rice, or pasta every day.

    b. Look for "whole" before the grain name on the list of ingredients.

    2. *Vegetables:* In case we haven't made it clear, vegetables truly are good for you! Do you remember when your mother used to say, "Eat your vegetables, they're good, and they're good for you"? She was right! To stay well, eat a lot of them; more as you grow older. Because needs change with age, we've added a chart from the Centers for Disease Control (CDC) to make it clear. If you're physically active, you may be able to eat even more and not gain weight. Eating vegetables daily helps prevent certain diseases, including some cancers, and helps control your weight. According to a study published in May 2009,[5] only 29.4 percent of Americans eat three to five servings of vegetables per day, and only 16.4 percent eat two to four servings of fruit per day. Eat your vegetables. They're good, and they're good for you.

TABLE 5.1 RECOMMENDED DAILY AMOUNT FOR VEGETABLES

	Age	Daily Recommendation
Children	2–3 years old	1 cup
	4–8 years old	1½ cups
Girls	9–13 years old	2 cups
	14–18 years old	2½ cups
Boys	19–13 years old	2½ cups
	14–18 years old	3 cups
Women	9–30 years old	2½ cups
	31–50 years old	2½ cups
	51+ years old	2 cups
Men	19–30 years old	3 cups
	31–50 years old	3 cups
	51+ years old	2½ cups

This table provides the Recommended Daily Amount (RDA) for vegetables; the table on the facing page further clarifies serving sizes.

How much is a cup of vegetables?[6] Serving sizes can be confusing—what is the difference between raw and cooked, for example? According to the CDC, 1 cup of raw or cooked vegetables or vegetable juice, or 2 cups of raw leafy greens, is equal to 1 cup from the vegetable group. Here is a chart that makes it clear:

TABLE 5.2 HOW MUCH IS A CUP OF VEGETABLES?

	Amount that counts as 1 cup of vegetables	Amount that counts as ½ cup of vegetables
DARK-GREEN VEGETABLES		
Broccoli	1 cup chopped or florets	3 spears, raw or cooked (5 inches long)
Greens (collards, mustard greens, turnip greens, kale)	1 cup, cooked	
Spinach	1 cup, cooked 2 cups raw = 1 cup vegetables	1 cup raw
ORANGE VEGETABLES		
Carrots	1 cup, strips, slices, or chopped, raw or cooked 2 medium-size 1 cup baby carrots (about 12)	1 medium-size carrot About 6 baby carrots
Pumpkin	1 cup mashed, cooked	
Sweet potato	1 large baked ≥ 2¼-inch diameter 1 cup sliced or mashed, cooked	
Winter squash (acorn, butternut, Hubbard)	1 cup cubed, cooked	
DRIED BEANS AND PEAS		
Dried beans and peas (such as black, kidney, pinto, soybeans, chickpeas, black-eyed peas, or split peas)	1 cup whole or mashed, cooked	
Tofu	1 cup ½-inch cubes (about 8 ounces)	1 piece 2½ by 2¾ by 1 inch (about 4 ounces)
STARCHY VEGETABLES		
Corn, yellow or white	1 cup 1 large ear (8 to 9 inches long)	1 small ear (about 6 inches long)
Green peas	1 cup	
White potatoes	1 cup diced, mashed French fried, 20 medium to long strips (2½ to 4 inches long)	1 medium-size, boiled or baked (2½- to 3-inch diameter)
OTHER VEGETABLES		
Bean sprouts	1 cup, cooked	
Cabbage, green	1 cup, chopped or shredded, raw or cooked	
Cauliflower	1 cup pieces or florets, raw or cooked	
Celery	1 cup, diced or sliced, raw or cooked 2 large ribs (11 to 12 inches long)	1 large rib (11 to 12 inches long)
Cucumbers	1 cup raw, sliced, or chopped	
Green or wax beans	1 cup, cooked	
Green or red bell peppers	1 cup chopped, raw, or cooked 1 large pepper (3-inch diameter, 3¾ inches long)	1 small pepper
Lettuce, iceberg or head	2 cups raw, shredded, or chopped	1 cup raw, shredded, or chopped
Mushrooms	1 cup raw or cooked	
Onions	1 cup chopped, raw or cooked	
Tomatoes	1 large raw whole (3-inch diameter) 1 cup, chopped or sliced, raw, canned, or cooked	1 small raw whole (1¼-inch diameter) 1 medium-size, canned
Tomato or mixed vegetable juice	1 cup	½ cup
Summer squash or zucchini	1 cup cooked, sliced or diced	

An easy (and fun) way to make sure you are getting the most from your veggies is to make sure there's a rainbow on your plate. The color chart below shows you how to eat a rainbow to get maximum benefit:[7]

TABLE 5.3 COLOR CHART OF FOOD: EAT A RAINBOW TO GET MAXIMUM BENEFIT

Food	Potential Benefit
RED	
Tomatoes (rich, red color from lycopene)	Prevent prostate cancer and cancers of the bladder, pancreas, and digestive tract
Peppers (hot and sweet)	Beta-carotene, vitamins C and A
Beets	Fiber, which helps reduce risk of heart disease and some cancers; folic acid; and vitamin C
ORANGE	
Winter squash, carrots, sweet potatoes, apricots, mangoes	Vitamin C, beta-carotene, antioxidants, which enhance the immune system
GREEN	
Spinach	Iron
Artichoke	Vitamin C and fiber
Broccoli, kale, collard greens, mustard greens	Calcium
Leafy vegetables	Vitamin A, folic acid
YELLOW	
Summer squash	Contains lutein, which may help prevent macular degeneration
Yellow pepper	Vitamin C
Pineapple	Manganese
PURPLE	
Red cabbage	High in antioxidants, rich in vitamins, high in fiber; contains indoles, nitrogen compounds that may help protect against breast cancer
Eggplant	Rich in nutrients, low in fat
WHITE	
Potatoes	Complex carbohydrates and B_6
Parsnips, onions, garlic, and cauliflower	High in vitamin C, fiber, allicin, and folic acid

TABLE 5.4 BENEFITS OF SELECTED VEGETABLES[1]

Nutrient	Benefit	Vegetable Sources
Fiber	Decreases risk of heart disease; regulates bowels	Navy beans, kidney beans, black beans, pinto beans, lima beans, white beans, soybeans, split peas, chickpeas, black-eyed peas, lentils, artichokes
Folate	Reduces risk of having a baby with a brain or spinal cord injury; reduces homocysteine levels, which can lower risk of blood clots; may reduce risk of colon polyps	Black-eyed peas, cooked spinach, great northern beans, asparagus
Potassium	Helps maintain healthy blood pressure	Sweet potatoes, tomato paste, tomato puree, beet greens, white potatoes, white beans, lima beans, cooked greens, carrot juice, prune juice
Vitamin A	Keeps eyes and skin healthy; helps protect against infections	Sweet potatoes, pumpkin, carrots, spinach, turnip greens, mustard greens, kale, collard greens, winter squash, cantaloupe, red peppers, Chinese cabbage
Vitamin C	Helps heal cuts and wounds and keeps teeth and gums healthy	Red and green peppers, kiwi, strawberries, sweet potatoes, kale, cantaloupe, broccoli, pineapple, Brussels sprouts, oranges, mangoes, tomato juice, cauliflower

1. Centers for Disease Control (CDC). "Fruit & Vegetable Benefits." Available at: www.fruitsandveggiesmatter .gov/benefits/ nutrient_guide.html (accessed July 20, 2009).

Red Hot Tip:

- Use fruits and/or vegetables to replace some of the other foods you're eating to unleash their power and reduce calories in your diet.
- Let off some steam! Steamed vegetables are delicious and low in calories. Steam until the color is bright and try not to overcook them.
- Use low-fat or low-calorie dressings to add flavor.
- If you boil vegetables, cut them into smaller pieces, ½ inch or smaller, to release their flavor quicker, within 20 minutes.
- Avoid breading and frying or high-fat dressings or sauces—they can add calories and fat to your diet, and actually diminish the fresh taste of vegetables!

3. *Fruits:*[8] Fruits are really good for you. They are a great source of vitamins, minerals, and fiber. Eat fruit as snacks and desserts. It doesn't matter if they are fresh, canned, frozen, or dried; they may be whole, cut up, or pureed. But remember to buy dried fruits that are processed without sugar. The whole fruit has much fewer calories than the fruit juice. Unlike vegetables, 1 cup of fruit or 100% fruit juice, or ½ cup of dried fruit is equal to 1 cup of fruit. Remember that some commercial fruit juices have added sweeteners, so make sure only to take the juices that are all natural.

How much fruit is needed daily? The amount of fruit you need to eat depends on age, sex, and level of physical activity. Recommended daily amounts are shown in table 5.5. Table 5.6, on the facing page, helps you to determine how much is a cup of fruit.

4. *Dairy:* Milk and foods made from milk are part of this food group. Foods such as cream cheese, cream, and butter lose the calcium from the milk, so they are not in this group.

Good examples are milk, yogurt, and cheese. Products that are low fat or fat free are best because you get the calcium but save a lot of the calories. Sweetened milk products have sugar added, so it

TABLE 5.5 RECOMMENDED DAILY AMOUNT FOR FRUIT*

	Age	Daily Recommendation
Children	2–3 years old	1 cup
	4–8 years old	1 to 1½ cups
Girls	9–13 years old	1½ cups
	14–18 years old	1½ cups
Boys	9–13 years old	1½ cups
	14–18 years old	2 cups
Women	19–30 years old	2 cups
	31–50 years old	1½ cups
	51+ years old	1½ cups
Men	19–30 years old	2 cups
	31–50 years old	2 cups
	51+ years old	2 cups

* These amounts are appropriate for individuals who get less than 30 minutes per day of moderate physical activity, beyond normal daily activities. Those who are more physically active may be able to consume more while staying within calorie needs. From CDC, http://www.mypyramid.gov/pyramid/fruits_amount_table.html.

adds extra calories to your diet. Many lactose-intolerant people can still eat hard cheeses and yogurt. Soy milk is another great lactose-free choice and can be used as a milk substitute. Soy comes in light versions that have even fewer calories. If you are lactose intolerant, you can also buy lactose-free cow's milk or use pills that have the lactase enzyme, so you can drink milk and milk products without side effects.

TABLE 5.6 HOW MUCH IS A CUP OF FRUIT?

	Amount that counts as 1 cup of fruit	Amount that counts as ½ cup of fruit
APPLE	½ large (3¼-inch diameter)	1 small (2½-inch diameter)
	1 cup, sliced or chopped, raw or cooked	½ cup, sliced or chopped, raw or cooked
APPLESAUCE	1 cup	
	1 (4-ounce) snack container	
BANANA	1 cup, sliced	
	1 large (8 to 9 inches long)	1 small (less than 6 inches long)
CANTALOUPE	1 cup, diced, or melon balls	
	1 medium-size wedge (⅛ medium-size melon)	
GRAPES	1 cup, whole or cut up	
	32 seedless grapes	16 seedless grapes
GRAPEFRUIT	1 medium-size (4-inch diameter)	½ medium (4-inch diameter)
	1 cup, sections	
MIXED FRUIT (FRUIT COCKTAIL)	1 cup, diced or sliced, raw or canned, drained	1 (4-ounce) snack container, drained ⅜ cup)
ORANGE	1 large (3-inch diameter)	
	1 cup, sections	1 small (2½-inch diameter)
ORANGE, MANDARIN	1 cup, canned, drained	
PEACH	1 large (2¾-inch diameter)	1 small (2-inch diameter)
	1 cup, sliced or diced, raw, cooked, or canned, drained	1 (4-ounce) snack container, drained (⅜ cup)
	2 halves, canned	
PEAR	1 medium size-pear (about 6 ounces)	1 (4-ounce) snack container, drained (⅜ cup)
PINEAPPLE	1 cup, chunks, sliced or crushed, raw, cooked, or canned and drained	1 (4-ounce) snack container, drained (⅜ cup)
PLUM	1 cup, sliced, raw, or cooked	
	3 medium-size or 2 large plums	
	1 large plum	
STRAWBERRIES	About 8 large berries	
	1 cup, whole, halved, or sliced, fresh or frozen	½ cup, whole, halved, or sliced
WATERMELON	1 small wedge (1 inch thick)	
	1 cup, diced, or melon balls	6 melon balls
DRIED FRUIT (RAISINS, PRUNES, APRICOTS, ETC.)	½ cup dried fruit	¼ cup dried fruit (1.5-ounce box raisins)
100% FRUIT JUICE (ORANGE, APPLE, GRAPE, GRAPEFRUIT, ETC.)	1 cup	½ cup

TABLE 5.7 CALCIUM, CALORIE, AND FAT CONTENT OF COMMON DAIRY FOODS

	Calcium (mg)	Calories	Fat (g)		Calcium (mg)	Calories	Fat (g)
MILK AND MILK BEVERAGES				**DESSERTS (CONTINUED)**			
Milk, whole, 1 cup	291	150	8	Ice cream (11% milk fat), 1 cup	176	270	14
Milk, low-fat (2%), 1 cup	297	120	5	Sherbet (2% fat), 1 cup	103	270	6
Milk, low-fat (1%), 1 cup	300	100	1	**OTHER GOOD SOURCES OF CALCIUM**			
Milk, skim, 1 cup	302	85	0	Almonds	75	165	16
Chocolate milk (1%), 1 cup	287	160	1	Broccoli, cooked, ½ cup	47	25	0
Buttermilk, 1 cup	285	100	2	Collard greens, cooked, ½ cup	179	30	0
CHEESES				Kale, cooked, ½ cup	90	20	0
American, 1 oz.	174	105	9	Salmon, pink, canned, with liquid and bones, 3 oz.	167	120	5
Cheddar, 1 oz.	204	115	9				
Cottage, low-fat (1%), 1 cup	155	160	2	Sardines, canned in oil, with liquid and bones, 3 oz.	371	175	9
Mozzarella, part-skim, 1 oz.	207	80	5				
Swiss, 1 oz.	272	105	8	Snap beans, cooked, ½ cup	31	18	0
YOGURT				Tofu, firm, raw, ¼ block	166	118	7.1
Plain, low-fat, 8 oz.	415	145	3	Curdled with calcium salt	553	118	7.1
Plain, nonfat, 8 oz.	452	125	0	Tofu, regular, raw, ¼ block	122	88	5.6
Fruit, low-fat, 8 oz.	345	230	3	Curdled with calcium salt	406	88	5.6
Coffee or vanilla, 8 oz.	389	194	3	Soybeans, dry roasted, ½ cup	232	387	18.6
DESSERTS				Soybeans, boiled, ½ cup	88	149	7.7
Ice milk, hardened, 1 cup	176	185	6	Soy protein concentrate, 1 oz.	102	93	0.13
Ice milk, soft serve, 1 cup	274	225	5	Soy milk, enriched, 1 cup	300	130	4

RECOMMENDED DAILY CALCIUM INTAKE

- 4- to 8-year-olds 1,000 mg/day
- 9- to 18-year-olds 1,550 mg/day
- Pregnancy/breast-feeding 1,200 mg/day
- Premenopausal adult 1,000 mg/day

- Postmenopausal:
  - Taking estrogen 1,000 mg/day
  - Not taking estrogen 1,500 mg/day

5. *Meat and Beans:* This part of the pyramid includes meat, poultry, fish, dried beans, eggs, and nuts.

PLANT FOODS RICH IN PHYTOESTROGENS

The word *phyto* means "plant." These so-called plant or *dietary* estrogens have a chemical structure similar to estrogen, so they work in the body like a weak estrogen. The major phytoestrogen groups are isoflavones (found mostly in soy), flavones, coumestans, and lignans (found mostly in flaxseeds). Here are some other foods that have phytoestrogens:

Hummus
Dried dates, apricots, and prunes
Sesame seeds
Winter squash
Multigrain bread
Black beans
Alfalfa sprouts
Yams
Garlic
Walnuts, chestnuts, and pistachios
Mung bean sprouts

Of course, it can feel pretty impossible to create a well-balanced meal all the time—there are always those moments when you want a snack. That's where smart snacks come in. When you get hungry during the day, instead of reaching for a candy bar or bag of cookies or chips, think fruits and vegetables. Here are some great choices recommended by the CDC that are about 100 calories or less and perfect for a Red Hot Mama snack:[9]

- 1 medium-sized apple (72 calories)
- 1 medium-sized banana (105 calories)
- 1 cup steamed green beans (44 calories)
- 1 cup blueberries (83 calories)
- 1 cup grapes (100 calories)
- 1 cup carrots (45 calories), broccoli (30 calories), or bell peppers (30 calories) with 2 tablespoons, hummus (46 calories)

SOME OTHER GOOD STRATEGIES AND REMINDERS

Six Red Hot Tips to Size Up Your Portion:[10]

1. Three ounces of meat is about the size and thickness of a deck of cards.
2. A medium-size apple or peach is the size of a tennis ball.
3. One ounce of cheese is the size of four dice.
4. A cup of broccoli is about the size of your fist.
5. One teaspoon of butter or peanut butter is the size of the tip of your thumb.
6. One ounce of nuts equals one handful.

UNDERSTANDING FOOD LABELS

Food labels can be confusing; here are the Food and Drug Administration (FDA) Guidelines for common food claims:

Low Calorie: <40 calories per serving

Low Cholesterol: <20 mg of cholesterol and 2 g of saturated fat per serving

Reduced: 25 percent less of the specified nutrient or calories than the usual product

Good source of: provides at least 10 percent of the daily value of a particular vitamin or nutrient per serving

Calorie free: Less than 5 calories per serving

Fat free/sugar free: <0.5 g of fat or sugar per serving

Red Hot Tips We've Learned from Yogis:[11]

- *Eat mindfully.* Eat slowly and experience your food; don't eat while watching TV and don't jump up immediately from the table when finished eating; relax a moment and digest.
- *Chew your food.* Digestion starts in your mouth and the more you chew your food the easier it will be to digest it. The yogis say, "There are no teeth in your stomach."
- *Listen to your body.* When you start to feel full, stop eating.
- *The "two-fist rule."* Make two fists with your hands and hold them in front of your stomach. This is the *total* amount of food you should have in your stomach at any one time. The yogic prescription for filling your stomach is one-third food, one-third water, and one-third space for digestion.
- *When to eat.* Eat your largest meal between 11 AM and 2 PM. Steamed vegetables or light vegetable salads are great choices for an evening meal. This helps prevent heartburn and acid reflux.
- *Eat a healthy snack.* Such as raisins and a few nuts or a banana in the late afternoon to keep your energy up and prevent overeating at dinner.

Low Sodium: <140 mg of sodium per serving

High in: provides at least 20 percent of the daily value of a specified nutrient per serving

High fiber: 5 or more grams of fiber per serving

RED HOT TIPS FROM DEAN ORNISH TO HELP HIGH-FAT RECIPES LOSE SOME FAT[12]

- Use nonfat sour cream or nonfat yogurt instead of sour cream for dressings and sauces. Avoid boiling after adding nonfat yogurt to prevent it from separating.
- Use liquid egg substitute with no added fat or egg whites instead of whole eggs for baking.
- Use fat-free vegetable broth, wine, or water instead of oil for sautéing onions and garlic, and simmer vegetables until tender.
- Use fat-free Italian dressing as a substitute for oil-and-vinegar dressing, or drizzle salads and vegetables with balsamic vinegar, raspberry vinegar, or tarragon vinegar.
- Use nonfat mayonnaise or yogurt instead of mayonnaise on sandwiches and in potato salad.

Whole-grain mustard alone is a great addition for flavor.

- Use prune puree or unsweetened applesauce instead of fat in baked goods. The puree is easy to make by whipping 4 ounces of pitted prunes and 5 tablespoons of water, or you can buy prepared fruit or prune puree, or use baby food. The ratio of prune puree to fat is 1:2. So, for ½ cup of butter, use ¼ cup of prune puree.
- Use nonfat sour cream or skim milk thickened with cornstarch instead of cream in pasta sauces. First dissolve cornstarch in a little cold water, using 1 tablespoon of cornstarch for each 1 cup of liquid you are replacing. You can also use 1 tablespoon of flour whisked into 1 cup of nonfat milk as an alternative substitute for heavy cream.

In addition to Dr. Ornish's excellent suggestions, here are a few of our favorite tips for substitutions to lose or control weight:

Whole eggs. Replace with liquid eggs or egg whites or a tablespoon of soy flour combined with 2 tablespoons of water.

For breakfast. Replace one of the eggs or half of the cheese in your omelet with spinach, onions, or mushrooms, or reduce the amount of cereal in your bowl and replace it with cut-up bananas, peaches, blueberries, or strawberries. Both add volume and flavor with fewer calories.

For lunch. Replace 2 ounces of the cheese and 2 ounces of the meat in your sandwich, wrap, or burrito with lettuce, tomatoes, cucumbers, or onions; replace 1 cup of noodles or 2 ounces of meat in your favorite broth-based soup with a cup of chopped vegetables, such as broccoli, carrots, beans, or red peppers.

For dinner. Replace 1 cup of the rice or pasta in your dish with 1 cup of chopped vegetables, such as tomatoes, squash, onions, peppers, or broccoli.

IN A NUTSHELL: FOODS TO AVOID—AND FOODS THAT MAY HELP IN MENOPAUSE MOMENTS

Hot flashes. Avoid spicy foods, large meals, hot beverages, and alcohol. Add soy foods (edamame, tofu, soy nuts) to your diet.

Mood swings. Avoid sugar blasts such as doughnuts, sweetened soda, and candy. They send your blood sugar up and down quickly and bring your mood with it. Foods rich in B vitamins, such as beets, Brussels sprouts, and asparagus, may help relieve depression.

Headaches. Stay away from alcohol and MSG (monosodium glutamate—often in Chinese foods), and start eating magnesium-rich foods such as almonds and black beans.

Achy joints. Stay away from caffeinated drinks that rob your body of calcium and eat foods rich in omega-3 fatty acids such as salmon, which may reduce those aches and pains.

Memory lapses. Skipping meals can affect your memory and concentration. Remember when your mom said, "You can't start your day on an empty stomach"? She was right again. Antioxidant-rich foods such as blueberries and vegetables help slow down those memory lapses.

THE RECIPES

Now that we've set the stage with the information you need on diet, nutrition, and exercise, it's time to set the table and serve up some delicious (and healthy) recipes to help you feel your best Red Hot Mama self. We've started in our own kitchens and then roamed far and wide—from the White House kitchen to the Black Dog Café on Martha's Vineyard; from the Fairmont in Chicago to the Flying Biscuit Café in Atlanta (former Hells Kitchen contestant); from Sydney, Australia, to Los Angeles and in between, all developed with an eye toward helping you be the hottest, healthiest, happiest Red Hot Mama you can be! And, guess what? Your family will benefit, too (and they won't even know they're eating health food!).

6

BREAKFAST

Strawberry-Yogurt Shake

This is a refreshing drink that is healthy and tastes great. It's perfect for at home or on the go.

Yield: 4 servings

½ cup unsweetened pineapple juice
¾ cup low-fat, plain yogurt
1½ cups frozen, unsweetened strawberries

Place the ingredients, in the order listed, into a food processor. Puree at medium speed until thick and smooth.

—Dr. Mache's Kitchen

Per serving: 118 Cal.; 42 GI; 3 g Prot.; 26 g Carb.; 0.4 g SFA; 0.2 g MUFA; 0.1 g PUFA; 0.05 g Omega-3; 112 mg Calc.; 34 mg Sod.; 426 mg Pot.; 1 mg Iron; 0 mg Phytoestrogen; 4 g Fiber

Soy Smoothie

This is a delicious breakfast, snack, or dessert that is rich in isoflavones, so it's good for hot flashes and building strong bones.

Yield: 2 servings (I cup each)

I cup vanilla or plain soy milk
I medium-size banana
¼ cup fresh or frozen unsweetened strawberries, or fresh or frozen unsweetened peaches (optional)
5 ice cubes (only if using fresh fruit)
I strawberry, for garnish

Place all the ingredients in a food processor and process on medium speed for 1 minute, or until smooth. Garnish with a strawberry and serve.

—Dr. Mache's Kitchen

Per serving: 129 Cal.; 71 GI; 5 g Prot.; 24 g Carb.; 0.3 g SFA; 0.4 g MUFA; 1 g PUFA; 0.6 g Omega-3; 158 mg Calc.; 71 mg Sod.; 395 mg Pot.; 1.5 mg Iron; 14 mg Phytoestrogen; 3 g Fiber

Maine Wild Blueberry Granola French Toast

Blueberries are chock-full of disease-fighting antioxidants. Toss some fresh ones on top for a treat. This dish is a great way to start off your day!

Yield: 2 servings

Batter:

2 eggs, separated

2 tablespoons sugar

¼ cup milk

French Toast:

2 (1-inch-thick) slices brioche toast

1 cup Wild Maine blueberry granola, ground coarsely

2 tablespoons butter

Preheat the oven to 450°F.

To make the batter, whip the egg whites until they form a soft peak, adding the sugar only at the end. In a separate bowl, whisk the yolks and the milk together. Gently fold one-third of the whites into the yolk mixture. Fold the remaining whites into the mixture in two separate stages.

To make the French toast, dip the toast slices into the batter to coat evenly. Sprinkle the tops evenly with the granola. Heat the butter in an ovenproof skillet over medium-high heat. Place the slices of toast in the skillet and cook for 4 to 5 minutes, until golden brown on the bottom, and then flip the toast slices over and place the pan in the oven for 3 to 4 minutes to finish cooking. Serve immediately with your favorite topping.

—Chef Jonathan Cartwright

Per serving: 468 Cal.; 62 GI; 15 g Prot.; 67 g Carb.; 3 g SFA; 8 g MUFA; 4 g PUFA; 0.7 g Omega-3; 115 mg Calc.; 334 mg Sod.; 310 mg Pot.; 3 mg Iron; 0.8 mg Phytoestrogen; 5 g Fiber

Whole-Grain Pancakes

This healthy recipe will soon become one of your favorites. These pancakes are heart healthy and better for diabetes than is a typical pancake mix. They are light and fluffy, and you can add blueberries or other fruits to your own unique taste.

Yield: 4 servings (2 pancakes per serving)

½ cup whole wheat flour

¼ cup sifted all-purpose flour

2 (3-tablespoon) scoops soy protein powder

2 teaspoons nonaluminum baking powder

¼ teaspoon salt

1⅓ cups soy milk or water

2 tablespoons oil

Cooking spray

Tip:

If you're looking for a simpler way to start your day, just reach into the food pantry, pull out your favorite pancake mix, and substitute soy milk in equal measure for the milk or water you would normally use.

Red Hot Ingredient: Whole Wheat

• Vitamins B and E
• Magnesium
• Fiber
• Antioxidants

Mix together the flours, soy protein powder, baking powder, and salt in a medium-size bowl. Add the soy milk and oil and stir just until blended. Spray a large skillet or griddle with cooking spray and heat over medium-high heat until hot enough to evaporate a drop of water immediately upon contact.

Spoon the batter by ¼-cup measures onto the hot pan. Cook until evenly covered with bubbles, about 2 minutes. Using a spatula, carefully turn over and cook for 1 to 2 minutes more, until lightly browned. Repeat with the remaining batter. Spray the pan again with cooking spray every time after making two pancakes.

—Dr. Mache's Kitchen

Per serving: 237 Cal.; 62 GI; 9 g Prot.; 32 g Carb.; 1 g SFA; 5 g MUFA; 3 g PUFA; 1 g Omega-3; 318 mg Calc.; 488 mg Sod.; 312 mg Pot.; 4 mg Iron; 9 mg Phytoestrogen; 3 g Fiber

Dewberry's Black Fingers Egg Scramble

This slightly spicy, rich breakfast scramble has more going for it than meets the eye. A delicious mix of eggs cooked with fingerling potatoes, black beans, garlic, and onions will start the day out right. You can top the finished scramble with diced tomatoes and avocado if you have them lying in wait. To reduce salt, use less Tabasco sauce. Enjoy!

Yield: I serving

5 or 6 small fingerling potatoes

I teaspoon extra-virgin olive oil

I to 2 tablespoons diced white onion

I clove garlic, minced

¼ to ⅓ cup canned black beans, drained and rinsed

2 eggs

½ teaspoon ground cumin

Salt and pepper

2 to 20 dashes Tabasco sauce

Diced tomato (optional)

Diced avocado (optional)

Place a few drops of water in a microwave-safe bowl. If your potatoes are thick, you will need to prick them with a fork before cooking. Place the potatoes in the bowl, cover with plastic wrap, and cook for 3 to 4 minutes on HIGH, or until the potatoes are tender. (Alternatively, peel the potatoes, place them in a pot of water, bring to a boil, and cook until tender.) Slice them in half and set aside.

In a stainless-steel saucepan, heat the olive oil over medium heat. Add the onion and sauté for 3 minutes. Add the potatoes and sauté for 1 minute longer. Add the garlic and sauté for another minute. Add the beans and sauté for 2 minutes more.

Break the eggs into a small bowl, add the cumin and salt and pepper to taste, and beat with a fork. Add to the bean mixture and cook for about 1 minute or more to your desired consistency.

Add as much Tabasco sauce as you like and top with the diced tomato and avocado if desired.

Per serving: 503 Cal.; 66 GI; 22 g Prot.; 58 g Carb.; 4 g SFA; 8 g MUFA; 2 g PUFA; 0.2 g Omega-3; 121 mg Calc.; 419 mg Sod.; 1,305 mg Pot.; 4 mg Iron; 0.19 mg Phytoestrogen; 10 g Fiber

—Jeffrey Parker

Eggs in the Nest

This recipe from the Low GI Family Cookbook *makes a lovely lazy weekend breakfast or brunch. Prepare double the quantity for four people—or for seconds. Use omega-3 eggs for less saturated fat, or egg whites.*

Yield: 2 servings

2 slices whole-grain bread

Olive oil cooking spray

1 teaspoon olive oil margarine

1½ ounces button mushrooms (about 4), stems trimmed, sliced

3 large (not baby) spinach leaves, washed and chopped

Freshly ground pepper

2 eggs

1 tablespoon coarsely grated reduced-fat Cheddar cheese

Preheat the oven to 350°F.

Cut the crusts off the bread. Spray both sides of each slice lightly with oil. Press the bread slices firmly into two ⅓-cup-capacity non-stick muffin cups. Set aside.

Heat the margarine in a nonstick skillet over medium-high heat until sizzling. Add the mushrooms and cook, stirring often, for 4 to 5 minutes, or until tender. Add the spinach and cook, stirring, for 1 to 2 minutes, or until wilted. Remove from the heat and season with pepper to taste.

Spoon half the mushroom mixture over each of the muffin cups of bread and press lightly. Crack an egg into a small dish and then slide it on top of the mushrooms. Repeat with the remaining egg and muffin cup. Sprinkle with the cheese. Bake for 15 minutes (for a softly set yolk), 20 minutes (for a hard-cooked yolk), or until the egg is cooked to your liking. Serve warm or at room temperature.

—*University of Sydney Glycemic Index and GI Database*

Per serving: 175 Cal.; 67 GI; 12 g Prot.; 13 g Carb.; 2 g SFA; 3 g MUFA; 1 g PUFA; 0.1 g Omega-3; 96 mg Calc.; 257 mg Sod.; 288 mg Pot.; 2 mg Iron; 0 mg Phytoestrogen; 2.5 g Fiber

Fresh Cranberry Muffins

These muffins are pretty special. Good for you and delicious, they are a great breakfast muffin for a traffic-laden commute. If fresh cranberries are out of season, use dried cranberries or raisins, but the muffin will be a lot sweeter and not nearly as tart.

Yield: 8 muffins

Raw sugar (optional)
¾ cup all-purpose flour
⅓ cup sugar
2 teaspoons baking powder
½ teaspoon baking soda
Pinch of salt
¾ teaspoon ground cinnamon
1 cup unprocessed miller's wheat bran
½ cup 1% milk
1 egg
2 tablespoons oil
½ cup chopped fresh cranberries

Preheat the oven to 400°F. Line eight standard muffin cups with paper baking cups. Sprinkle very lightly with raw sugar if desired.

In a medium-size mixing bowl, combine the flour, sugar, baking powder, baking soda, salt, cinnamon, and wheat bran and mix well. In another bowl, combine the milk, egg, oil, and cranberries and mix well. Make a well in the center of the dry ingredients and pour in the wet ingredients. Mix just until combined, using as few strokes as possible.

Fill the muffin cups about three-quarters full with the batter and bake for 10 to 20 minutes, until a toothpick inserted in the center comes out clean.

—Jeffrey Parker

Per serving: 100 Cal.; 65 GI; 3 g Prot.; 16 g Carb.; 0.5 g SFA; 2 g MUFA; 1 g PUFA; 0.3 g Omega-3; 96 mg Calc.; 281 mg Sod.; 128 mg Pot.; 1.5 mg Iron; 0 mg Phytoestrogen; 4 g Fiber

Breakfast to Go

For a mild and delicious stimulant, this is clearly "the way to go," thanks to the high fiber in prunes.

Yield: I serving

12 almonds (with skins)

6 pitted prunes

Soak the almonds and the pitted prunes overnight in 1 cup of water. In the morning, blend the mixture in a food processor until liquefied as completely as possible. Drink as a morning drink. (Don't be surprised if the almonds have begun to sprout after 6 hours of soaking.)

—*Dr. Mache's Kitchen*

> **Red Hot Ingredient: Prunes**
>
> • Vitamin A
> • Magnesium
> • Fiber

Per serving: 222 Cal.; 29 GI; 4 g Prot.; 40 g Carb.; 0.6 g SFA; 4.5 g MUFA; 2 g PUFA; 0.01 g Omega-3; 64 mg Calc.; 1 mg Sod.; 522 mg Pot.; 1 mg Iron; 0 mg Phytoestrogen; 6 g Fiber

7

APPETIZERS AND SIDE DISHES

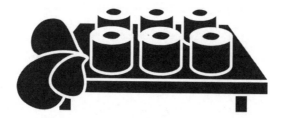

Mock Chopped Liver

I love chopped liver, but it doesn't love me. It contains lots of saturated fats and calories and proves the point that everything that tastes good isn't good for you. Then Bubbie came up with "Mock" Chopped Liver to keep the taste and the tradition going and win the hearts of her guests without clogging their hearts' arteries. This recipe is low in sodium and saturated fat, high in fiber, and an excellent source of protein as well.

Yield: 3 to 4 cups

4 medium-size onions, sautéed

4 hard-boiled eggs

1 (17-ounce) can chickpeas, drained and rinsed

½ cup walnuts, chopped

Salt and pepper

Blend all ingredients in a food processor or in a chopping bowl. Serve a scoop of the "chopped liver" on a lettuce leaf.

—*Bubbie's Kitchen*

Per serving: 287 Cal.; 46 GI; 14 g Prot.; 30 g Carb.; 2 g SFA; 4 g MUFA; 6 g PUFA; 1 g Omega-3; 79 mg Calc.; 157 mg Sod.; 423 mg Pot.; 3 mg Iron; 0 mg Phytoestrogen; 7 g Fiber

Spinach, Basil, and Red Pepper Wraps

Chef Goldfarb has combined delightful flavors and fresh vegetables to make one of the best wraps in the world. Peppers are vitamin rich and their beta-carotene may help preserve eye health.

Yield: 4 servings

4 large whole wheat or flour tortillas

8 teaspoons mango chutney or honey mustard

24 leaves fresh basil

8 slices reduced-fat Cheddar cheese

1 red bell pepper, seeded, ribs removed, and cut into long, thin strips

4 cups baby spinach, washed well

Heat the tortillas in a microwave (alternatively, some people prefer to heat them over an open flame on the stovetop for a few seconds) until they are warm and soft.

Spread 2 teaspoons of the mango chutney or honey mustard on one side of each tortilla. Top the spread on each wrap with six basil leaves, placed from one end to the other. Top the basil with two slices of cheese, one-quarter of the red bell pepper (lay the strips across the middle of the tortilla so you can roll it up), and 1 cup of the spinach.

Roll the wraps as tightly as possible, and slice them in half or into bite-size pieces before serving.

—Aviva Goldfarb

Per serving: 355 Cal.; 48 GI; 16 g Prot.; 25 g Carb.; 7 g SFA; 6 g MUFA; 1 g PUFA; 0.3 g Omega-3; 376 mg Calc.; 667 mg Sod.; 397 mg Pot.; 2 mg Iron; 0 mg Phytoestrogen; 4 g Fiber

Red Hot Ingredient: Peppers

• Vitamins A, B_1, B_6, C, and K, and folic acid
• Beta-carotene
• Fiber
• Antioxidants

To Lose or Control Weight . . .

Replace 2 ounces of the cheese and 2 ounces of the meat in your sandwich, wrap, or burrito with lettuce, tomatoes, cucumbers, or onions.

Goat Cheese Monte Cristo

In the quest to eat healthier, more and more people have become interested in goat cheese. Goat cheese is highly nutritious and great for most women who are lactose intolerant.

Yield: 14 sandwiches

1 brioche loaf

½ pound soft goat cheese, crumbled

½ pound aged goat cheese (drunken goat cheese), grated

1½ to 2 cups chopped mixed fresh herbs (e.g., parsley, chives, chervil, thyme)

Salt and pepper

14 slices Serrano ham

All-purpose flour

2 eggs, lightly beaten

Panko

Oil, for deep-frying

Thinly slice the brioche into twenty-eight slices. Combine the cheeses, herbs, and salt and pepper to taste in a mixing bowl. Spread the cheese mixture on fourteen slices of the brioche, and then place a slice of ham on top of the cheese and dust with the flour.

Brush with the beaten eggs and sprinkle with the panko. Cover the sandwich halves with the remaining slices of brioche.

Heat the oil in a deep skillet and deep-fry the sandwiches, a few at a time, turning them over to brown on each side.

Set aside to drain on paper towels. Serve hot.

—*Chef Neal Fraser*

Per serving: 181 Cal.; 67 GI; 10 g Prot.; 10 g Carb.; 7 g SFA; 3 g MUFA; 0.5 g PUFA; 0.02 g Omega-3; 188 mg Calc.; 188 mg Sod.; 68 mg Pot.; 1.5 mg Iron; 0 mg Phytoestrogen; 0.5 g Fiber

Nori Rolls

Nutritious nori is a good wrap for party hors d'oeuvres. These rolls also make a great meal when served with salad greens and grilled shiitake mushrooms. The magnesium in avocado may help with sleep.

Yield: 25 nori rolls

5 sheets nori

2½ cups cooked brown rice (1 cup brown rice cooked in 1¾ cups water yields 2½ cups cooked rice)

2½ teaspoons wasabi paste, or wasabi powder, diluted according to package directions

1 avocado, peeled, pitted, and cut into small cubes

1 cucumber, peeled, julienned, and cut into 1-inch lengths

3 carrots, peeled, julienned, and cut into 1-inch lengths

5 green onions, julienned and cut into 1-inch lengths

Place a sheet of nori on a bamboo sushi-rolling mat. Moisten your hands with water and spread ¾ cup of brown rice evenly over the surface of the nori sheet, leaving bare a 1½-inch-wide strip along the top edge. Spread ½ teaspoon of the wasabi paste over about one-third of the sheet, parallel with the top edge, and place a strip each of the vegetables on top. Starting at the bottom, roll the nori sheet, wrapping the vegetables, toward the top, using steady pressure. You may need to moisten the edge slightly to seal.

Repeat with the remaining nori, rice, wasabi, and vegetables.

Wrap each roll in plastic wrap and refrigerate until serving. To serve, cut each roll with a sharp knife into five pieces.

—*Benay Vynerib*

Per serving: 113 Cal.; 50 GI; 3 g Prot.; 19 g Carb.; 0.4 g SFA; 2 g MUFA; 0.5 g PUFA; 0.03 g Omega-3; 30 mg Calc.; 266 mg Sod.; 279 mg Pot.; 1 mg Iron; 0 mg Phytoestrogen; 5 g Fiber

Red Hot Ingredient: Avocado

- B vitamins and vitamin E
- Calcium, magnesium, and potassium
- Monounsaturated fatty acids
- Fiber

Red Hot Ingredient: Nori

- Vitamins A, B_2, and C
- Magnesium and potassium

Caribbean-Style Black Bean and Rice Salad

Easy to prepare, this lovely appetizer can also be served as a luncheon dish. Chopped, cooked, and cooled shrimp makes a wonderful omega-3-rich addition to this recipe. Fat free and filling, black beans keep blood sugar levels low after a meal, making them a good choice for people with diabetes.

Yield: 6 to 8 servings

Dressing:

½ cup olive oil

¼ cup white wine vinegar

1 tablespoon Dijon mustard

1 tablespoon ground cumin

1 tablespoon minced garlic

Salt and pepper

Beans and Rice:

1 (15-ounce) can black beans, drained and rinsed

2½ cups cooked white rice (1 cup white rice cooked in 1¾ cups water yields 2½ cups cooked rice), cooled

¾ cup seeded and chopped red bell pepper

¾ cup seeded and chopped yellow bell pepper

¾ cup chopped green onion

Salt and pepper

To make the dressing, whisk the olive oil, vinegar, mustard, cumin, and garlic in a small bowl until well blended. Season to taste with salt and pepper.

To make the salad, combine the beans, rice, peppers, and green onion in a large bowl. Toss the salad with enough dressing to moisten and season with salt and pepper to taste.

—*Cynthia Niles*

Per serving: 273 Cal.; 55 GI; 6 g Prot.; 30 g Carb.; 2 g SFA; 10 g MUFA; 2 g PUFA; 0.22 g Omega-3; 52 mg Calc.; 255 mg Sod.; 316 mg Pot.; 2.3 mg Iron; 0.3 mg Phytoestrogen; 7 g Fiber

Red Hot Ingredient: Black Beans

• Fiber
• Protein
• Antioxidants

Stuffed Zucchini

Get your RDA of veggies with this easy-to-prepare recipe, which uses an abundant—and abundantly nutritious—summer vegetable.

Yield: 8 servings

2 medium-large zucchini

3 to 4 slices whole wheat bread, diced small

½ cup reduced-fat shredded sharp Cheddar cheese

½ teaspoon salt

¼ teaspoon pepper

¼ teaspoon dried oregano

⅛ teaspoon garlic powder

3 tablespoons olive oil

Red Hot Ingredient: Zucchini

- Vitamins A and C, and folic acid
- Potassium
- Lutein

Preheat the oven to 425°F. Lightly grease a medium-size baking dish.

Trim both ends of each zucchini, slice in half lengthwise, and cut each slice in half crosswise. Place the zucchini pieces in a large saucepan with water and parboil until tender but not mushy. Drain and cool, and then scoop out and discard the seeds.

Combine the bread, cheese, salt, pepper, oregano, garlic powder, and olive oil in a large bowl. Mix well and stuff into the hollow of each piece of zucchini. Place the zucchini in the greased baking dish and bake for 15 minutes. Serve hot.

—*Cynthia Niles*

Per serving: 209 Cal.; 68 GI; 7 g Prot.; 16 g Carb.; 3 g SFA; 8 g MUFA; 1 g PUFA; 0.1 g Omega-3; 120 mg Calc.; 368 mg Sod.; 374 mg Pot.; 1 mg Iron; 0.05 mg Phytoestrogen; 3 g Fiber

Black Bean Salsa

Yes, salsa is a vegetable! This is a wonderful salsa for a buffet, and it can be prepared in a jiffy. Serve chilled.

Yield: 6 to 8 servings

1 (15-ounce) can black beans, rinsed and drained

1 red bell pepper, seeded and cut into small bite-size pieces

1 green bell pepper, seeded and cut into small bite-size pieces

1 red onion, cut into small bite-size pieces

½ cup chopped fresh cilantro

½ cup balsamic vinegar

2 tablespoons crushed garlic

2 tablespoons freshly squeezed lime juice

Salt and pepper

In a large mixing bowl, combine the beans, peppers, onion, and cilantro. In small mixing bowl, whisk together the vinegar, garlic, lime juice, and salt and pepper to taste, and then pour over the black bean mixture and toss to mix well. Chill in the refrigerator and serve with tortilla chips.

—*Cynthia Niles*

Per serving: 56 Cal.; 40 GI; 2 g Prot.; 11 g Carb.; 0.03 g SFA; 0.04 g MUFA; 0.15 g PUFA; 0.05 g Omega-3; 28 mg Calc.; 113 mg Sod.; 170 mg Pot.; 1 mg Iron; 0 mg Phytoestrogen; 3 g Fiber

Tip: Cocktail party advice

If you are going to a cocktail party, always eat something solid before you get there so you won't go overboard on the appetizers.

Sesame Tamari Tofu

Easy to make, this delicious dish is rich in phytoestrogens, which may help with hot flashes and bone health. High-protein tofu may also decrease LDL (bad) cholesterol, which may reduce our risk for heart disease

Yield: 4 servings

Cooking spray

1 (15-ounce) package firm or extra-firm tofu

2 tablespoons tamari

1 tablespoon crushed or whole sesame seeds

2 green onions, chopped

Preheat the oven to 350°F. Spray a medium-size baking dish with cooking spray.

Slice the tofu into ten to twelve slabs and put them in a gallon-size sealable plastic bag. Add the tamari; seal the bag, squeezing out any air; and turn to coat the tofu evenly. Refrigerate for at least 15 to 20 minutes, turning the bag occasionally.

Place the tofu in the prepared baking dish and sprinkle with the sesame seeds. Bake for 20 to 25 minutes, or until lightly browned, turning once or twice for even browning. Top with the green onions and serve hot.

—Hari Kaur Khalsa

Per serving: 115 Cal.; 23 GI; 11 g Prot.; 3.5 g Carb.; 0.7 g SFA; 5 g MUFA; 1 g PUFA; 0 g Omega-3; 213 mg Calc.; 458 mg Sod.; 184 mg Pot.; 2.5 mg Iron; 24 mg Phytoestrogen; 1 g Fiber

Edamame

A classic sushi bar snack, edamame is a natural remedy for hot flashes and keeping bones strong, and it is an excellent source of protein. A great food for Red Hot Mamas!

Yield: 4 servings

½ pound soybeans in the pod
⅛ teaspoon salt

Place the soybeans in a medium-size saucepan and add 2 cups of water to cover. Bring to a boil over high heat and boil for 10 to 15 minutes. Drain and chill in the refrigerator. Arrange the beans in a fanned-out pattern on a serving platter and sprinkle with salt. Diners can shell the beans themselves as they eat them. (The pods are inedible.)

—Dr. Mache's Kitchen

Per serving: 80 Cal.; 50 GI; 7 g Prot.; 6 g Carb.; 0.4 g SFA; 0.6 g MUFA; 2 g PUFA; 0.2 g Omega-3; 82 mg Calc.; 79 mg Sod.; 306 mg Pot.; 1 mg Iron; 10 mg Phytoestrogen; 2.3 g Fiber

What Are Phytoestrogens?

Phytoestrogens are plant foods that have a chemical structure similar to estrogen, so they work in the body like a weak estrogen. The major phytoestrogen groups are isoflavones (found mostly in soy), flavones, coumestans, and lignans (found mostly in flaxseeds).

Roasted Soy Nuts

Although they seem like peanuts, soy nuts are actually roasted whole soybeans. They make a great healthy snack.

Yield: 4 servings

1 cup shelled fresh soybeans
Cooking spray
⅛ teaspoon salt

Red Hot Ingredient: Soybeans

- Vitamin C
- Calcium and iron
- Protein
- Isoflavones
- Omega-3 and omega-6 fatty acids

Place the soybeans in a medium-size bowl, cover with 2 cups of water, and soak for about 3 hours. (Choose a bowl that will allow the beans to double in size.)

Preheat the oven to 350°F and spray a cookie sheet with cooking spray.

Drain and spread the soybeans on the prepared cookie sheet and roast for about 45 minutes, until browned, stirring every 10 to 15 minutes.

Lightly salt to taste and store in an airtight container. They should keep for a month at room temperature.

—Dr. Mache's Kitchen

Per serving: 105 Cal.; 15 GI; 9 g Prot.; 8 g Carb.; 0.7 g SFA; 1 g MUFA; 3 g PUFA; 0.3 g Omega-3; 33 mg Calc.; 123 mg Sod.; 317 mg Pot.; 1 mg Iron; 30 mg Phytoestrogen; 4 g Fiber

Pan-Seared Sardines, Slow-Cooked Grains, Swiss Chard, Golden Raisins, Pine Nuts, and Smoked Paprika

This dish may have a lot of ingredients, but the combination is fantastic—well worth it not only for the flavor, but a great dose of omega-3s! One caveat: This recipe does contain a lot of salt. Consider substituting reduced-sodium chicken broth.

Yield: 4 servings

Slow-Cooked Grains and Swiss Chard:
⅔ cup wheat berries or bulgur
2 tablespoons extra-virgin olive oil
1 cup chopped Vidalia onion
2 cloves garlic, minced
1 leaf lemon thyme, chopped
3 quarts chicken broth
½ cup French lentils or any other kind of lentils
1½ cups chopped red Swiss chard
Pinch of ground cinnamon
2 tablespoons chopped fresh cilantro
1 teaspoon salt
1 teaspoon freshly ground pepper

Pan-Seared Sardines:
12 sardines (3 ounces each without heads, guts, and scales) or any other fish high in omega-3 fats, such as salmon or mackerel
1 tablespoon extra-virgin olive oil
Salt and pepper

To make the slow-cooked grains and Swiss chard, soak the wheat berries in 1 quart of water overnight. The next day, heat the olive oil in a large, heavy saucepan and sauté the onion, garlic, and lemon thyme until the vegetables are tender. Add the wheat berries and chicken broth to the saucepan and bring to a boil over high heat. Lower the heat and simmer, covered, for about 25 minutes. Add the lentils and more chicken broth if necessary and continue to simmer, covered, for 12 more minutes. Add the chard and cook, covered, for another 5 minutes, and then stir in the cinnamon, cilantro, salt, and pepper. Cover and set aside on the stove top to keep warm.

To make the pan-seared sardines, drizzle the sardines with the olive oil and sprinkle with a pinch of salt and pepper. Preheat a large skillet until it turns very hot. Add the sardines and cook them for about 1½ minutes on each side. Transfer the sardines to a bowl and set aside. Do not wash out the skillet.

Pan-Seared Sardines, Slow-Cooked Grains, Swiss Chard, Golden Raisins . . . (continued)

Golden Raisins, Pine Nuts, and Smoked Paprika:

4 tablespoons extra-virgin olive oil

¼ cup golden raisins

2 tablespoons pine nuts

8 small grape tomatoes, halved

1 tablespoon white balsamic vinegar or any white wine vinegar

1 tablespoon chopped Italian parsley

1 teaspoon smoked Spanish paprika or any other paprika

Salt and pepper

Garnishes:

Chopped parsley

Freshly ground pepper

Cilantro sprigs

Whole-Grain Goodness

When grains are "refined," it means that the bran and germ portions of the grain kernel have been removed. This also means that the fiber has been removed. If you do eat refined grains, make sure they are enriched, meaning the makers put back in the B vitamins and iron that are removed during the refining process. The fiber in whole grains helps you eat more slowly and fill up naturally, and this helps prevent overeating. Ideally, it's best to stick with whole grains!

To make the golden raisins, pine nuts, and smoked paprika, using the same skillet (unwashed) as the sardines were cooked in, heat the olive oil over medium heat and add the raisins, pine nuts, and tomatoes and sauté for 1 minute. Turn the heat off and stir in the vinegar, parsley, paprika, and salt and pepper to taste.

To serve, warm four individual serving plates. Spoon a portion of the hot grains mixture onto each plate and top each with three sardines. Pour the sautéed raisin mixture over the sardines. Garnish each serving with the chopped parsley and a few grindings of pepper and decorate each with a few sprigs of cilantro. Serve hot.

—Chef Luis Bollo

Per serving (slow-cooked grain and Swiss chard): 360 Cal.; 42 GI; 24 g Prot.; 40 g Carb.; 2 g SFA; 7 g MUFA; 2 g PUFA; .15 g Omega-3; 70 mg Calc.; 3,836 mg Sod.; 1,083 mg Pot.; 5 mg Iron; 0 mg Phytoestrogen; 9 g Fiber

Per serving (pan-seared sardines): 95 Cal.; 0 GI; 9 g Prot.; 0 g Carb.; 1 g SFA; 3 g MUFA; 2 g PUFA; 1 g Omega-3; 5 mg Calc.; 20 mg Sod.; 226 mg Pot.; .4 mg Iron; 0 mg Phytoestrogen; 0 g Fiber

Per serving (raisins, pine nuts, and smoked paprika): 183 Cal.; 60 GI; 1 g Prot.; 9 g Carb.; 2 g SFA; 11 g MUFA; 3 g PUFA; .1 g Omega-3; 10 mg Calc.; 4 mg Sod.; 154 mg Pot.; 1 mg Iron; 0 mg Phytoestrogen; 1 g Fiber

Stuffed Bell Peppers

Stuffed peppers are a great meal that won't leave you feeling stuffed. These are a delicious, low-saturated-fat approach for meat eaters in the family, and go great with brown rice and a salad. For many people, one pepper half is just the right portion size, but two will satisfy even hearty eaters. Be sure to include red bell peppers, for more than just their color—they have significantly higher levels of nutrients than green.

Yield: 8 servings

5 bell peppers (red, yellow, green, orange), halved and seeded

1 tablespoon canola oil

1 large onion, chopped

1 pound lean ground turkey

2 tablespoons cooked brown rice

1 (8-ounce) and 1 (15-ounce) can tomato sauce

Salt and pepper

Preheat the oven to 350°F.

Place the ten bell pepper halves facing up in a 9 by 13-inch baking dish.

Heat the canola oil in a small skillet over medium heat. Add the onion and sauté until the onion is tender. In a mixing bowl, combine the turkey, sautéed onions, rice, 8-ounce can of tomato sauce, and a pinch each of pepper and salt and mix well. Stuff the peppers with the meat mixture. Pour the 15-ounce can of tomato sauce over the peppers and cover the baking dish with aluminum foil. Place in the oven and bake for 1½ hours.

—*Dr. Mache's Kitchen*

Per serving: 144 Cal.; 53 GI; 14 g Prot.; 11 g Carb.; 1 g SFA; 2 g MUFA; 1 g PUFA; 0.2 g Omega-3; 27 mg Calc.; 465 mg Sod.; 517 mg Pot.; 2 mg Iron; 0 mg Phytoestrogen; 2 g Fiber

Eggplant Pakoras

This is a popular Indian dish that contains lots of good vegetables and seasonings. It can be served with a salad for a delicious, light meal. Eggplant is low in calories but super nutritious.

Yield: 4 to 6 servings

1 teaspoon dried oregano

½ teaspoon ground cinnamon

2 teaspoons turmeric

1 teaspoon freshly ground pepper

½ teaspoon ground cloves

2 teaspoons salt

1 tablespoon caraway seeds

1 teaspoon cardamom seeds

2 cups chickpea flour

¾ cup onion juice or puree

½ cup milk

¼ cup honey

Vegetable oil or ghee, for frying

1 eggplant, cut crosswise into ⅜-inch slices

In a large mixing bowl, combine the spices, salt, and seeds with the chickpea flour and mix well. Add the onion juice, milk, ⅓ cup of water, and the honey and stir into a paste, mixing with a fork until smooth.

Heat the oil in a large skillet over medium-high heat. Dip the eggplant slices in the batter and fry them until golden brown. Transfer to paper towels to drain. Serve with ketchup or chutney.

—*Hari Kaur Khalsa*

Per serving: 222 Cal.; 58 GI; 9 g Prot.; 41 g Carb.; 0.5 g SFA; 1 g MUFA; 1 g PUFA; 0.1 g Omega-3; 88 mg Calc.; 819 mg Sod.; 609 mg Pot.; 3 mg Iron; 1 mg Phytoestrogen; 8 g Fiber

Red Hot Ingredient: Eggplant

- Many B-complex vitamins
- Copper, iron, manganese, and potassium
- Nasunin (an antioxidant)
- Fiber

Couscous with Pumpkin, Almonds, and Dried Apricots

A versatile alternative to rice, couscous is quick and easy to cook.

Yield: 6 servings

4 tablespoons olive oil

2 cups pumpkin, peeled, seeded, and diced small

1 tablespoon brown sugar

Salt

1 cup minced yellow onions

2 cloves garlic, minced

¼ teaspoon ground cinnamon

Pinch of ground cloves

3 cups chicken broth

2 cups couscous

3 tablespoons finely chopped fresh mint

¼ teaspoon finely chopped fresh rosemary

½ cup chopped Marcona almonds

½ cup dried apricots, sliced thinly

Red Hot Ingredient: Pumpkin

- Vitamin A
- Beta-carotene
- Fiber

Red Hot Ingredient: Couscous

- B-complex vitamins, especially niacin
- Selenium
- Fiber

Preheat the oven to 375°F.

In a large bowl, mix 2 tablespoons of the olive oil with the pumpkin and brown sugar and season to taste with salt.

Spread on a baking sheet and bake in the oven for 20 minutes.

Heat the remaining 2 tablespoons of the olive oil in a saucepan over medium-high heat. Add the onion and sauté for 5 minutes. Add the garlic and sauté for 2 minutes more.

Add the cinnamon and cloves and sauté for 1 minute longer.

Add the chicken broth and heat through.

Place the couscous in a large metal bowl. Pour the hot broth mixture over the couscous. Wrap the whole bowl with plastic wrap and let sit for 10 minutes. Remove the plastic wrap and fluff the couscous with a fork. Fold in the mint, rosemary, almonds, and apricots. Season as needed and serve.

—*Michelle Bernstein*

Per serving: 650 Cal.; 57 GI; 20 g Prot.; 92 g Carb.; 3 g SFA; 15 g MUFA; 4 g PUFA; 0.14 g Omega-3; 108 mg Calc.; 278 mg Sod.; 804 mg Pot.; 3 mg Iron; 0 mg Phytoestrogen; 9 g Fiber

Kasha

Kasha is a staple food in many Eastern European cuisines. It's versatile, inexpensive, and easy to prepare. The high protein in buckwheat is not digested, which allows it to absorb cholesterol from food and prevent it from being absorbed by the intestines. It works great both as a light meal when served with a salad or as a side dish.

Yield: 6 servings

1½ cups raw kasha (medium-size buckwheat groats)

2 eggs

3 cups boiling water

½ tablespoon salt

4 tablespoons heart-healthy buttery spread

1 onion, diced

Red Hot Ingredient: Buckwheat

• B-complex vitamins
• Protein

Preheat the oven to 350°F.

Place the kasha in a shallow baking dish or pie pan. Stir in, but do not beat, the eggs until the kasha is coated. Bake with the oven door slightly ajar, until the grains are dry (about 25 minutes). Shake the pan and stir the kasha about every 5 minutes to keep the groats from sticking. Transfer the kasha to a large saucepan. Add the boiling water and salt. Cover and cook over moderate heat for 10 to 15 minutes. It may be necessary to add a little more water. (When done, the kasha will be tender and doubled in bulk, and all the cooking water absorbed.)

Heat the buttery spread in a skillet over medium-high heat. Add the onion and sauté until browned, and then scrape the onion and butter into the kasha, stir, and serve.

—*Bubbie's Kitchen*

Per serving: 194 Cal.; 46 GI; 6 g Prot.; 22 g Carb.; 6 g SFA; 3 g MUFA; 1 g PUFA; 0.06 g Omega-3; 22 mg Calc.; 475 mg Sod.; 136 mg Pot.; 1 mg Iron; 0 mg Phytoestrogen; 3 g Fiber

Green Bean Bits with Crispy Garlic

Fresh from your garden or a local market, green beans are a refreshing vegetable side dish any time of year and are loaded with fiber (4 grams per cup). When they are paired with crispy garlic and mild olive oil, you will be reaching for a guilt-free second helping of this dish! Select the deep green, crunchy beans for best results.

Yield: 5 servings

1 pound fresh regular or French green beans

5 to 6 cloves garlic, sliced thinly

2 tablespoons mild-flavored oil (such as canola oil, or even olive oil)

Salt and pepper

Cut the green beans into ¾-inch lengths. The easiest way to do this is to grab a handful, line them up, and slice through the bunch.

Heat the oil in a skillet over medium-high heat. Add the garlic and a pinch of salt and sauté very carefully, until the garlic is golden; be very careful not to let it burn. When the garlic is golden, add the beans and sauté until they are tender and slightly blistered, about 5 minutes. Serve and enjoy!

—Joanne Choi

Per serving: 82 Cal.; 60 GI; 2 g Prot.; 8 g Carb.; 0.5 g SFA; 3 g MUFA; 1.5 g PUFA; 0.5 g Omega-3; 40 mg Calc.; 242 mg Sod.; 204 mg Pot.; 1 mg Iron; 0 mg Phytoestrogen; 3 g Fiber

Mashed Sweet Potatoes and Apples

This recipe is a tasty alternative to traditional mashed or baked potatoes, and it goes well with roast chicken, turkey, or pork. Sweet potatoes are fat free and packed with nutrients that help our metabolism and may prevent the development of heart disease and cancer.

Yield: 8 servings

2 pounds sweet potatoes (about 6 medium-size), left whole and unpeeled

1 tablespoon plus 1½ teaspoons butter

½ cup chopped onion

2 large Granny Smith apples, peeled, cored, and chopped coarsely (2½ cups)

¼ teaspoon salt

¼ teaspoon freshly ground pepper

¼ teaspoon grated nutmeg

Garnish:
Chopped dill or parsley

Red Hot Ingredient: Sweet Potatoes

- Vitamins A, B, and C
- Calcium and iron
- Beta-carotene
- Carotenoids
- Fiber

Bring a large saucepan of water to a boil over high heat. Add the whole sweet potatoes and boil briskly for 30 to 35 minutes, or until tender. Drain and let cool slightly.

In a large skillet with a lid, melt the 1 tablespoon of butter over medium heat. Add the onion and cook, stirring occasionally, for 6 to 8 minutes, or until golden and tender. Add the apples and 2½ tablespoons of water and cook, covered, over medium-low heat for 10 to 15 minutes, or until the apples are tender.

Preheat the oven to 375°F and grease a medium-size baking dish.

Peel the potatoes (the skin should slip off), cut into chunks, and put into a large bowl. Add the 1½ teaspoons of butter, salt, pepper, nutmeg, and the apple mixture and mash with a potato masher or the back of a spoon until smooth. Spoon the mixture into the greased baking dish and bake for 25 to 30 minutes.

Garnish with dill or parsley and serve.

—Cynthia Niles

Per serving: 181 Cal.; 45 GI; 2 g Prot.; 37 g Carb.; 2 g SFA; 1 g MUFA; 0 g PUFA; 0 g Omega-3; 49 mg Calc.; 160 mg Sod.; 434 mg Pot.; 1 mg Iron; 0 mg Phytoestrogen; 5 g Fiber

Carrot-Pineapple Slaw

A new way to prepare slaw, this recipe would complement any meal nicely. Grandma was right: Carrots really do keep our eyes healthy.

Yield: 6 servings (I cup each)

I cup diced fresh pineapple or drained canned pineapple chunks, juice reserved

½ cup raisins

I (10-ounce) package matchstick-cut carrots

2 tablespoons canola oil

2 tablespoons freshly squeezed lemon juice

2 tablespoons maple syrup

I tablespoon fresh pineapple juice (if you use canned pineapple, you can use the juice from the can)

2 tablespoons chopped Italian (flat-leaf) parsley

¼ teaspoon salt

⅛ teaspoon freshly ground pepper

Combine the pineapple, raisins, and carrots in a large bowl. In a small bowl, combine the canola oil, lemon juice, maple syrup, and pineapple juice and whisk until well blended. Pour the oil mixture over the pineapple mixture and toss well. Add the parsley, salt, and pepper and toss well. Cover and chill before serving.

—Cynthia Niles

Per serving: 194 Cal.; 60 GI; 1.5 g Prot.; 34 g Carb.; 0.5 g SFA; 4 g MUFA; 2 g PUFA; 0.6 g Omega-3; 53 mg Calc.; 203 mg Sod.; 485 mg Pot.; 1 mg Iron; 0 mg Phytoestrogen; 3 g Fiber

Red Hot Ingredient:
Carrots

- Vitamin A
- Beta-carotene
- Fiber

8

SOUPS AND STEWS

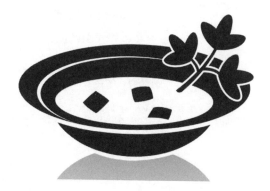

Crab and Sweet Potato Soup

This soup is a never-ending delight that you can enjoy year-round. Low-fat, low-carb crabmeat and sweet potatoes are a winning combination.

Yield: 6 to 8 servings

2 pounds sweet potatoes, peeled and diced

½ yellow onion, diced

4 cloves garlic, minced

1 tablespoon ground coriander

1 teaspoon salt

1 teaspoon grated nutmeg

½ teaspoon cayenne

½ teaspoon ground white pepper

2 whole cloves

1½ cups dry sherry

1 cup orange juice

¼ cup lemon juice

1 tablespoon hoisin sauce

1 pound crabmeat (claw)

Combine all the ingredients except the crab with 8 cups of water in a large saucepan. Cover and bring just to a boil over medium-high heat, and then lower the heat and simmer, covered, for 20 to 30 minutes, until the potatoes are tender. Puree the soup in a food processor or with an immersion blender and return to the saucepan. Add the crabmeat and heat through. Serve hot.

—*Chef Tres Hundertmark*

Per serving: 235 Cal.; 50 GI; 14 g Prot.; 30.5 g Carb.; 0.2 g SFA; 0.2 g MUFA; 0.5 g PUFA; 0.3 g Omega-3; 116 mg Calc.; 382 mg Sod.; 564 mg Pot.; 2 mg Iron; 0.2 mg Phytoestrogen; 3.3 g Fiber

Red Hot Ingredient: Crabmeat

- Vitamins A and C
- Calcium, copper, iron, magnesium, phosphorous, and zinc
- Protein
- Amino acids

Maine Fiddlehead Fern Soup

This wonderful and unusual soup can be enjoyed in the spring, when fiddlehead ferns are in season. Fiddlehead ferns are fat, cholesterol, and sodium free and have been eaten for centuries in Australia, New Zealand, and Asia.

Yield: 4 servings

3 tablespoons butter*
1 onion, chopped
1 clove garlic, minced
1 pound fiddleheads
2 teaspoons salt
White pepper
4 cups vegetable broth
1 cup milk
4 teaspoons crème fraîche

* To reduce the saturated fat content in this recipe, a heart-healthy buttery spread and low-fat milk can be used.

Red Hot Ingredient: Fiddlehead ferns

- Vitamins A, B$_3$, and C
- Iron and potassium

Melt the butter in a saucepan over medium-high heat. Add the onion, garlic, and fiddleheads and sauté until the onions are translucent and liquid has started to leach out of the vegetables. Sprinkle with the salt and a few grindings of white pepper. Add the vegetable broth and bring to a boil. Once boiling, add the milk and bring to a boil again. Remove from the heat and blend the soup in a high-speed bar blender or a food processor until smooth. Return to the saucepan, season to taste, and heat through. Pour into four individual soup bowls, top each with a teaspoon of crème fraîche, and serve.

—Chef Jonathan Cartwright

Per serving: 178 Cal.; 54 GI; 7 g Prot.; 15 g Carb.; 6 g SFA; 3 g MUFA; 0.4 g PUFA; 0.04 g Omega-3; 129 mg Calc.; 1,103 mg Sod.; 572 mg Pot.; 2 mg Iron; 0 mg Phytoestrogen; 3 g Fiber

Iced Watermelon and Maine Blueberry Soup

This tasty soup is perfect for a luncheon on a warm summer day, followed by a green salad and a light dessert. It's not only delicious, but healthy as well. Rich in potassium and lycopene, watermelon may also help reduce the risk of developing kidney stones.

Yield: 4 servings

1 (2-pound) watermelon

1 pound Maine blueberries

2 cups muscat or any sweet dessert wine, or orange juice

2 cups champagne, chilled

Peel, dice, and seed the watermelon. In a liquidizer or food processor, blend the watermelon, blueberries, and wine until smooth. Strain through a fine strainer and chill. Just before serving, add the chilled champagne.

—Chef Jonathan Cartwright

Per serving: 311 Cal.; 57 GI; 2 g Prot.; 29 g Carb.; 0 g SFA; 0 g MUFA; 0.1 g PUFA; 0 g Omega-3; 40 mg Calc.; 16 mg Sod.; 420 mg Pot.; 1 mg Iron; 0 mg Phytoestrogen; 2 g Fiber

To see a video of the song "Fruits Are Really Good for You," go to www .YouTube/com/HealthRockTV.

Fruits are really good for you. They are a great source of vitamins, minerals, and fiber.

Eat fruits as snacks and desserts. It doesn't matter if they are fresh, canned, frozen, or dried (remember to buy dried fruits that are processed without sugar). Enjoy whole, cut up, or pureed. Whole fruit has much fewer calories than fruit juice.

Roasted Sweet Potato and Apple Soup

This soup evokes images of oak furniture and a roaring fireplace at an old country inn. Sweet potatoes have lots of complex carbohydrates, which help keep our blood sugar balanced.

Yield: 6 servings (about 1½ cups each)

2 medium-size sweet potatoes, peeled and cut into medium-size chunks

1 firm apple, such as Gala or Jonagold, peeled, cored, and quartered

1 medium-size yellow onion, peeled and quartered

2 cloves garlic

2 tablespoons olive oil

Salt and pepper (optional)

3 to 4 cups low-sodium chicken or vegetable broth

¾ cup nonfat sour cream for serving (optional)

Variation:

Add ¼ to ½ teaspoon of ground ginger or 1 tablespoon of fresh grated ginger to the roasted vegetables before blending, or ¼ to ½ teaspoon of ground chipotle chile pepper for a spicy bite.

Preheat the oven to 450°F.

Put the sweet potatoes, apples, onion, and garlic in a roasting pan. Toss them with the olive oil and a few shakes of salt and pepper to taste, if using. Place in the oven and roast, tossing every 10 minutes, until the vegetables and apples are tender, about 30 minutes.

Add just enough broth to cover the mixture and puree in a food processor (or in the roasting pan, using an immersion blender). Add more broth if necessary to reach a consistency that is smooth and not too thick. (If you are using a food processor, you will probably need to puree the soup in two batches.)

Warm the soup over low heat in a saucepan until ready to serve, or refrigerate for up to 1 day or freeze for up to 3 months. Stir in the sour cream at the table for a creamier taste, if desired.

—*Aviva Goldfarb*

Per serving: 145 Cal.; 54 GI; 4 g Prot.; 23 g Carb.; 0.6 g SFA; 3 g MUFA; 0.5 g PUFA; 0.03 g Omega-3; 71 mg Calc.; 427 mg Sod.; 353 mg Pot.; 1 mg Iron; 0 mg Phytoestrogen; 2 g Fiber

Rocky Mountain Minestrone

This delicious Italian-style minestrone soup is filled with hearty and healthy vegetables and beans. It makes a great inexpensive family meal or side dish. Often soup is based on the strength of the broth being used. If you don't use homemade, a good-quality canned stock will suffice. If you use store-bought broth, it can be salty, so season accordingly or use sodium-reduced broth. Cabbage is low in calories and high in fiber.

Yield: 6 main-dish servings or 12 side-dish servings

3 tablespoons extra-virgin olive oil

1 large white onion, chopped

¼ cup all-purpose flour

1 cup dry sherry or dry red wine

2 large potatoes, peeled and cut into ½-inch cubes

1 small head white cabbage, cored and chopped into bite-size pieces

2 ribs celery, chopped

2 zucchini, cut into ½-inch cubes

2 large tomatoes, chopped

1 cup cooked white beans (you can use canned, but home cooked is better)

1 cup cooked chickpeas (you can use canned, but home cooked is better)

Chicken or vegetable broth

Salt and pepper

1 teaspoon chopped fresh basil, or ¼ teaspoon dried

1 bay leaf

½ bunch of fresh Italian (flat-leaf) parsley, chopped

½ pound pasta shells or 1 cup raw rice (optional)

Garnish:
Extra-virgin olive oil or pesto

Heat the olive oil in a large saucepan over medium heat. Add the onion and sauté until translucent but not browned. Whisk in the flour to make a roux (this is for thickening). To the saucepan, add the sherry, potatoes, cabbage, celery, zucchini, tomatoes, and beans (drain and rinse the beans first, if using canned). Add enough broth to cover and bring to a boil, skimming off any froth that rises to the surface. Once all the froth has been skimmed off, lower the heat to low and add salt and pepper to taste (remember, you can add more, but you can't take it out, so season as you go). Add the basil, bay leaf, and parsley and simmer, covered, until the vegetables are tender but not mushy.

Rocky Mountain Minestrone (continued)

Red Hot Ingredient: Cabbage

- Vitamin C
- Potassium
- Beta-carotene
- Fiber

When the vegetables are done, add the pasta or rice if desired, and cook until al dente. Before serving, drizzle the top of each serving with extra-virgin olive oil or 1 tablespoon of pesto.

—Antonio Laudisio

Per serving: 525 Cal.; 54 GI; 16 g Prot.; 87 g Carb.; 1 g SFA; 5 g MUFA; 2 g PUFA; 0.15 g Omega-3; 129 mg Calc.; 670 mg Sod.; 1,133 mg Pot.; 5 mg Iron; 0.2 mg Phytoestrogen; 11 g Fiber

Tip:

Buy organic broths even though they may be a wee bit more expensive; they will have a lot more flavor. Also, if you use low-sodium broths, it allows you to season your soup yourself.

Lentil Soup

Italians eat lentils on New Year's, as soon after midnight as possible. The lentils symbolize coins and are supposed to help bring prosperity in the new year. Lentils are also a good source of protein and they also contain many trace minerals. The large amount of fiber in lentils is effective in lowering cholesterol and managing blood sugar disorders. With just 230 calories for a whole cup of cooked lentils, they will fill you up—not out.

Yield: 4 servings

1 teaspoon salt
2¼ cups lentils
3 carrots, pared and chopped
2 ribs celery, chopped
1 onion, chopped finely
¼ cup extra-virgin olive oil
1 clove garlic, peeled
1 ounce anchovy fillets in oil, drained
1 (16-ounce) can tomatoes, chopped
Salt and pepper
Handful of torn fresh basil
Handful of chopped fresh Italian (flat-leaf) parsley
Extra-virgin olive oil, for drizzling

Red Hot Ingredient: Lentils

- Vitamin B$_1$ and folic acid
- Iron
- Protein
- Cysteine and methionine (amino acids)
- Fiber

Put 6 cups of water and the salt in an 8-quart saucepan. Add the lentils, carrots, celery, and onion and cook over medium heat for 10 minutes.

In a separate large saucepan, warm the olive oil over low heat. Add the garlic clove and cook until it becomes golden brown. Remove the garlic and add the anchovies, tomatoes, and salt and pepper to taste. Stir in the basil.

Drain the lentils and reserve the cooking water. Pour the lentils into the tomato mixture, gradually adding enough cooking water to make a thick soup. Cook over medium heat until the lentils are al dente (about 30 minutes).

Sprinkle the parsley over the soup, drizzle a small amount of olive oil over the top, and serve.

—*Karen's Cucina*

Per serving: 494 Cal.; 24 GI; 32 g Prot.; 75 g Carb.; 1 g SFA; 6 g MUFA; 2 g PUFA; 0.3 g Omega-3; 151 mg Calc.; 478 mg Sod.; 1,661 mg Pot.; 12 mg Iron; 0 mg Phytoestrogen; 21 g Fiber

Angel Hair Pasta, Chickpea, Escarole, and Sausage Soup

A steamy bowl of this highly flavorful soup will comfort you the entire day. Escarole is chock-full of healthy nutrients that exert antioxidizing and powerfully health-promoting effects on the body. For a lower-sodium version, use sodium-reduced beef broth.

Yield: 4 servings

3 tablespoons extra-virgin olive oil

½ cup chopped onion

1 rib celery, chopped

2 tablespoons chopped fresh rosemary

2 medium-size Italian sweet sausages, casings removed and meat crumbled

4 cups beef broth

1 (15-ounce) can chickpeas, drained and rinsed

1 small head escarole, washed and chopped

Pinch of crushed red pepper flakes

4 cloves garlic, sliced thinly

4 tablespoons tomato paste

4 ounces angel hair pasta, broken into 1-inch pieces

Salt and pepper

Freshly grated Parmesan cheese

Heat the olive oil in a large saucepan over medium heat. Add the onion, celery, and rosemary and sauté for 8 minutes.

Then add the sausage and sauté until browned. Add the broth, 3 cups of water, and the chickpeas, escarole, red pepper, garlic, and tomato paste and bring to a boil over medium-high heat, and then lower the heat and simmer, covered, for 25 minutes. Add the pasta and simmer, covered, for an additional 10 minutes, just until the pasta is al dente.

Add salt and pepper to taste. Serve garnished with the freshly grated Parmesan cheese.

—Karen's Cucina

Per serving: 564 Cal.; 45 GI; 25 g Prot.; 63 g Carb.; 6 g SFA; 13 g MUFA; 4 g PUFA; 0.3 g Omega-3; 131 mg Calc.; 1,759 mg Sod.; 856 mg Pot.; 6 mg Iron; 2 mg Phytoestrogen; 10 g Fiber

Red Hot Ingredient: Escarole

- Vitamins A, C, and K, and folic acid
- A host of phytonutrients

Chicken Soup with Pasta

This is a great soup recipe with a beautiful blend of homemade chicken broth and vegetables that are in perfect harmony with the pasta. Chicken soup has long been touted to relieve cold and flu symptoms. The beta-carotene in the carrots helps enhance white blood cells to fight infections, and the onions are also strong antioxidants. Chilling the soup after cooking and skimming off the layer of congealed fat from the top can make the soup relatively low fat.

Yield: 4 servings

1 (3½-pound) broiler-fryer chicken with its giblets

2 medium-size carrots, pared

1 large parsnip, pared

1 onion

2 ribs celery

2 celery tops

3 sprigs of fresh Italian (flat-leaf) parsley

1 leek

1 tablespoon salt

12 peppercorns

3 cups acini di pepe pasta (or substitute orzo or other small pasta, such as annellini, ditalini, or tubettini)

Freshly grated Parmesan cheese

Per serving: 857 Cal.; 52 GI; 97 g Prot.; 57 g Carb.; 6 g SFA; 8 g MUFA; 6 g PUFA; 0.4 g Omega-3; 109 mg Calc.; 501 mg Sod.; 1,163 mg Pot.; 7.5 mg Iron; 0 mg Phytoestrogen; 6 g Fiber

In a large casserole, combine the chicken, giblets, carrots, parsnip, onion, and celery. Tie the celery tops, parsley, and leek together with kitchen string and add to casserole. Add enough cold water to cover the chicken and vegetables. Heat slowly to boiling, skimming off any froth that rises to the surface.

Add the salt and peppercorns, lower the heat, and simmer, covered, for 1½ hours, until the meat starts to fall off the bones. Remove the meat and vegetables from the broth and discard the bundle of greens that were tied with string. When cool enough to handle, take the meat off the bones, chop the vegetables, and put the chicken and vegetables back into the broth.

In a saucepan, cook the pasta al dente according to the package instructions. Drain the pasta and add it to the chicken soup. Serve topped with freshly grated Parmesan cheese.

—Karen's Cucina

Red Hot Mamas Minestrone Soup

Mmmmm . . . nothing better than minestrone soup for a Red Hot Mama. This is a simple, satisfying soup stocked with fresh vegetables. Eating this soup is a great way to include healthy vegetables and legumes in your diet.

Yield: 4 servings

1 (3-pound) shin of beef
1 tablespoon salt
5 carrots, pared
2 ribs celery, chopped
1 onion, quartered
5 sprigs of fresh Italian (flat-leaf) parsley
1 bay leaf
1 (16-ounce) can tomatoes
1 (20-ounce) can chickpeas, undrained
1 (10-ounce) package frozen cut green beans
1 (10-ounce) package frozen peas
2 cups chopped cabbage
¼ pound spaghetti, broken into 1-inch pieces
Salt and pepper

Place the shin of beef, salt, and 4 quarts of water in a large saucepan.

Cover and bring to a boil, skimming off any froth that rises to the surface. Lower the heat and add the carrots, celery, onion, parsley, and bay leaf. Simmer, uncovered, for 3 hours. Remove the beef and carrots and set aside. Strain the broth (there should be about 8 cups). In the same saucepan, combine the broth, tomatoes, chickpeas, green beans, peas, cabbage, spaghetti, and salt and pepper to taste. Bring to a boil, then lower the heat and simmer, covered, for 45 minutes.

Meanwhile, slice the carrots and remove the beef from the bone and add to the simmering soup near the end of cooking. Serve hot.

—*Karen's Cucina*

Per serving: 950 Cal.; 46 GI; 107 g Prot.; 91 g Carb.; 5 g SFA; 6 g MUFA; 3 g PUFA; 0.1 g Omega-3; 239 mg Calc.; 725 mg Sod.; 1,937 mg Pot.; 16 mg Iron; 2 mg Phytoestrogen; 19 g Fiber

Red Hot Ingredient: Chickpeas

• Folic acid
• Copper, iron, magnesium, manganese, and zinc
• Protein
• Fiber

Pasta and Bean Soup (Pasta e Fagioli)

Pasta e fagioli is a real comfort soup, and also provides iron, fiber, magnesium, folate, and thiamine. There are a tremendous number of local variations of this soup in Italy. This particular version is one of Karen's favorite family recipes from Sicily.

Yield: 4 servings

¼ cup extra-virgin olive oil

3 cloves garlic, minced

1 onion, chopped

1 rib celery, diced

3 tablespoons tomato paste

⅓ cup pancetta, chopped

6 tablespoons minced fresh rosemary

½ teaspoon dried basil

Salt and pepper

2 cups canned chicken broth

2 cups canned cannellini beans, drained and rinsed

½ pound pasta

½ cup freshly grated Parmigiano-Reggiano cheese

Heat the olive oil in a large saucepan over medium-low heat. Add the garlic, onion, celery, tomato paste, pancetta, rosemary, basil, and salt and pepper to taste and sauté for 8 minutes. Add the broth and bring it to a boil, then lower the heat and simmer, covered, for 10 minutes. Add the beans and simmer, covered, for another 15 minutes.

In a separate pot, cook the pasta al dente according to the package instructions, drain, and add to the soup. If the soup is too thick, add a little water. Add salt and pepper to taste and serve topped with the freshly grated cheese.

—*Karen's Cucina*

Per serving: 607 Cal.; 42 GI; 28 g Prot.; 75 g Carb.; 5 g SFA; 12 g MUFA; 2.5 g PUFA; 0.2 g Omega-3; 284 mg Calc.; 1,442 mg Sod.; 897 mg Pot.; 6 mg Iron; 0.2 mg Phytoestrogen; 9 g Fiber

Piquillo Pepper and Tomato Soup

This inventive soup is excellent, and a cup of it is the great start to a great meal.

Yield: 8 to 10 servings

1 (16-ounce) can plum tomatoes

1 (16-ounce) can Roma tomatoes

¼ cup butter (½ stick)

½ cup chopped yellow onion

1 large carrot

2 cloves garlic

2 teaspoons smoked paprika

6 canned piquillo peppers, or 2 small whole roasted red bell peppers

8 cups chicken broth

Pinch of saffron

Salt and pepper

Preheat the oven to 350°F.

Put the tomatoes in a roasting pan and roast for about 1 hour, or until slightly charred.

In a large, heavy-bottomed saucepan, heat the butter over medium-high heat. Add the onions and sauté until tender. Add the carrots, garlic, and paprika and sauté until the vegetables are tender. Stir in the charred tomatoes and peppers, and then pour in the chicken broth. Lower the heat and simmer, covered, for 2 hours. When the soup is cooked, blend it in a food processor. Strain the soup through a fine strainer, return it to the saucepan, and then stir in the saffron and season it with salt and pepper to taste. Heat through and serve.

—Chef Neal Fraser

Per serving: 190 Cal.; 52 GI; 12 g Prot.; 18 g Carb.; 4 g SFA; 3 g MUFA; 2 g PUFA; 0.2 g Omega-3; 105 mg Calc.; 690 mg Sod.; 570 mg Pot.; 4 mg Iron; 0 mg Phytoestrogen; 5 g Fiber

Chilled Tomato Soup

This wonderful cold soup is easy to prepare and it has an abundance of flavors, plus the antioxidant protection of lots of tomatoes. This recipe not only will be delicious to your taste buds but it will also help keep you healthy.

Yield: 8 servings

9 vine-ripe tomatoes, peeled, seeded, and diced

1 medium-size red onion, diced

5 cloves garlic, crushed

¼ cup chopped fresh marjoram

½ cup red wine vinegar

2 teaspoons ground cumin

2 teaspoons ground coriander

2 teaspoons yellow curry powder

2 teaspoons paprika

3 cups tomato juice

Salt and pepper

½ cup olive oil

1 tablespoon sugar

In a large bowl, combine the tomatoes, onion, garlic, marjoram, vinegar, cumin, coriander, curry powder, paprika, and tomato juice. Cover and let marinate for 3 hours. Whisk in the oil and sugar and then blend in a food processor until smooth. Chill for 4 hours before serving.

—*Chef Brad Parsons*

Per serving: 318 Cal.; 49 GI; 3 g Prot.; 17 g Carb.; 4 g SFA; 20 g MUFA; 3 g PUFA; 0.2 g Omega-3; 65 mg Calc.; 260 mg Sod.; 785 mg Pot.; 2 mg Iron; 0.1 mg Phytoestrogen; 4 g Fiber

Red Hot Ingredient: Tomatoes

- Vitamins A, B_2 and B_6, C, E, and K
- Chromium, copper, iron, manganese, and potassium
- Beta-carotene
- Lycopene
- Tryptophan (an amino acid)
- Fiber

The "Good" Cholesterol

HDL is considered the "good" cholesterol because it protects you from having a heart attack. It's different from the other cholesterol levels; the higher your HDL, the better. Several things can help you increase your HDL level: Quit smoking, lose excess weight, eat a good diet, and exercise. It's simple—healthy lifestyle changes can increase your HDL and decrease your risk of heart attack.

Borscht (Beet Soup)

If you're hot, eat it cold. If you're cold, eat it hot. Either way it's delicious, either before a meal or with a salad for a refreshing light meal on its own. The amino acid in beets, betaine, has been studied as having possible anticancer properties.

Yield: 10 servings

I small head green cabbage, shredded

2 potatoes, cut into I- to 2-inch cubes

4 medium-size ribs celery, diced

I onion, diced

I red or green bell pepper, seeded and diced

½ teaspoon salt

I teaspoon canola oil

4 beets, trimmed, peeled, and shredded

2 carrots, shredded

I (15-ounce) can tomato sauce

5 to 6 cloves garlic, minced

Fat-free sour cream for garnish

Red Hot Ingredient: Beets

- Vitamins A and C, biotin, folic acid, and niacin
- Calcium, magnesium, and manganese
- Betaine (an amino acid)
- Fiber

Place the cabbage, potatoes, celery, onion, and bell pepper in a large, heavy saucepan. Add 5 quarts of water and salt and bring to a boil over high heat. Lower the heat to medium and cook for about 45 minutes, or until the vegetables are tender.

Meanwhile, heat the canola oil in a medium-size saucepan over medium-high heat. Add the beets and carrots and sauté briefly.

Lower the heat to medium, add enough water to cover, and cook for 20 minutes. Add the tomato sauce, mix well, and add this mixture to the cabbage mixture, stirring well to combine.

Continue to cook over medium heat for 50 minutes longer. Add the garlic to the borscht and cook for 5 more minutes. Allow to cool to room temperature, and then place in a large container and refrigerate. Serve cold to cool hot flashes. Garnish each serving with 1 tablespoon of fat-free sour cream.

—*Dr. Mache's Kitchen*

Per serving: 61 Cal.; 58 GI; 2 g Prot.; 14 g Carb.; 0 g SFA; 0 g MUFA; 0 g PUFA; 0 g Omega-3; 52 mg Calc.; 180 mg Sod.; 458 mg Pot.; 1 mg Iron; 0 mg Phytoestrogen; 4 g Fiber

Mushroom-Barley Soup

This meatless adaptation of the classic soup tastes wonderful and is so healthy. Serve it with a green salad that has celery, walnuts, and feta cheese, with a loaf of warm sour-dough bread. Mushrooms have been eaten for thousands of years and also used for medicinal purposes.

Soup yield: 6 servings (2 cups each)

⅔ cup pearl barley (use quick-cooking barley or soak the barley in water overnight to cut cooking time)

8 cups reduced-sodium chicken or vegetable broth

2 tablespoons olive oil

1 yellow onion, chopped

1 teaspoon minced garlic (about 2 cloves)

2½ to 3 cups sliced mushrooms

2 ribs celery, sliced thinly

3 carrots, peeled and sliced thinly

1 tablespoon Worcestershire sauce

2 tablespoons dry sherry, or 1 tablespoon balsamic vinegar (optional)

¼ teaspoon salt, or to taste

⅛ teaspoon freshly ground pepper, or to taste

Rinse the barley in cold water (or drain the presoaked barley).

Combine the broth and barley in a large saucepan and bring it to a boil. Lower the heat and simmer, covered, stirring occasionally, until it is almost tender. (Note: If you are using quick-cooking barley, it should be tender after 10 minutes; presoaked barley should be tender after 20 minutes. If you haven't presoaked the barley, then simmer it for 40 minutes.)

Meanwhile, in a large heavy skillet heat the olive oil over medium-high heat. Add the onion and sauté until lightly browned, about 5 minutes. Add the garlic, mushrooms, and celery and sauté until the mushrooms are tender and have turned dark, about 5 more minutes.

Red Hot Ingredient: Barley

• Vitamin B_2 and niacin
• Copper, iron, magnesium, phosphorous, selenium, and zinc
• Fiber

Mushroom-Barley Soup (continued)

Variation:

Use the optional sherry and serve the soup with a hot pepper sauce, such as Tabasco.

Side dish salad suggestion: To make the salad, combine 6 cups of chopped iceberg or other lettuce; 2 ribs of celery, sliced; 2 tablespoons of chopped walnuts; and 2 tablespoons of crumbled feta cheese. Toss the salad with 2 to 4 tablespoons of dressing, such as homemade Maple-Dijon Dressing. (To make Maple-Dijon Dressing, whisk together ¼ cup of olive oil, ⅛ cup of red wine vinegar, 1 tablespoon of pure maple syrup, 1 teaspoon of Dijon mustard, and ½ teaspoon of herbes de Provence or dried thyme.)

Side dish bread suggestion: Warm a loaf of sourdough bread in a 300°F oven for 5 minutes.

After the barley has simmered for 10 to 40 minutes (see note above), add the mushroom mixture, carrots, and Worcestershire sauce to the barley. Simmer, covered, for 10 to 15 minutes, until the barley and carrots are tender. Stir in the sherry (optional, but highly recommended) and warm the soup through. Season the soup with salt and pepper to taste and serve immediately or freeze it for up to 3 months.

—*Aviva Goldfarb*

Per serving: 179 Cal.; 43 GI; 8 g Prot.; 26 g Carb.; 0.7 g SFA; 3 g MUFA; 0.7 g PUFA; 0.05 g Omega-3; 53 mg Calc.; 795 mg Sod.; 605 mg Pot.; 2 mg Iron; 0 mg Phytoestrogen; 5 g Fiber

Per serving (side salad): 148 Cal.; 50 GI; 3 g Prot.; 10 g Carb.; 2 g SFA; .7 g MUFA; 2 g PUFA; 0.4 g Omega-3; 64 mg Calc.; 74 mg Sod.; 382 mg Pot.; 1 mg Iron; 0 mg Phytoestrogen; 3 g Fiber

Per serving (sourdough bread): 370 Cal.; 61 GI; 15 g Prot.; 72 g Carb.; 0.6 g SFA; .4 g MUFA; 1 g PUFA; 0.06 g Omega-3; 56 mg Calc.; 832 mg Sod.; 164 mg Pot.; 5 mg Iron; 0 mg Phytoestrogen; 3 g Fiber

Fish Stew

This is a mouthwatering and succulent Italian fish stew that can be served year-round. Fish provides an excellent source of omega-3 fatty acids, vitamins, and minerals that benefit our general health. The American Heart Association recommends at least two servings of fish per week to help prevent heart disease, lower blood pressure, and reduce the risk of heart attacks and strokes. The rest of the ingredients are equally healthy, so eat up and feel great!

Yield: 4 servings

⅓ cup extra-virgin olive oil

1 onion, chopped

6 cloves garlic, sliced thinly

1 rib celery, chopped

1 carrot, peeled and chopped

1 (28-ounce) can tomatoes, chopped

1 cup dry white wine

½ pound cod, cut into bite-size pieces

½ pound snapper, cut into bite-size pieces

½ pound large shrimp, peeled and deveined

1 teaspoon dried oregano

Handful of fresh Italian (flat-leaf) parsley, chopped

Salt and pepper

Heat the olive oil in a large saucepan over medium heat. Add the onion, garlic, celery, and carrot and sauté for 8 minutes.

Add the tomatoes and wine and bring to a boil, then lower the heat and simmer, covered, for 30 minutes. Add the cod and snapper and simmer, covered, for an additional 15 minutes.

Then add the shrimp and simmer, covered, for another 5 minutes. Stir in the oregano, parsley, and salt and pepper to taste. If the stew is too thick, add a little water. Serve immediately.

—*Karen's Cucina*

Per serving: 336 Cal.; 54 GI; 24 g Prot.; 15.5 g Carb.; 3 g SFA; 13 g MUFA; 3 g PUFA; 0.6 g Omega-3; 110 mg Calc.; 402 mg Sod.; 876 mg Pot.; 3 mg Iron; 0 mg Phytoestrogen; 3 g Fiber

Vegetable Stew

This has become one of my favorite recipes. It's delicious, low caloric, and oh-so-good for you. It's a delicious way to get your daily recommended dose of veggies either as a side dish or an entrée. It's even better heated up the next day.

Yield: 4 to 6 servings

2 tablespoons canola oil

2 onions, chopped

2 to 3 carrots, sliced

1 summer squash, sliced

1 eggplant, peeled and sliced

1 zucchini, sliced

1 (8-ounce) package of mushrooms, sliced

1 cup cut fresh green beans (cut into 2-inch lengths)

1 (15-ounce) can tomato sauce

1 tablespoon ketchup

3 cloves garlic, minced

Salt and pepper

Grated Parmesan cheese, for garnish (optional)

Heat the canola oil in a large saucepan over medium heat. Add the onions, carrots, squash, eggplant, zucchini, mushrooms, and beans and cook, stirring occasionally, for about 30 minutes, or until the vegetables are tender. Lower the heat to low, then stir in the tomato sauce and ketchup and cook for 15 minutes.

Stir in the garlic and salt and pepper to taste and serve garnished with the Parmesan cheese if desired.

—*Dr. Mache's Kitchen*

Per serving: 193 Cal.; 57 GI; 7 g Prot.; 30 g Carb.; 0.6 g SFA; 4 g MUFA; 2 g PUFA; 0.7 g Omega-3; 77 mg Calc.; 598 mg Sod.; 1,358 mg Pot.; 2 mg Iron; 0 mg Phytoestrogen; 10 g Fiber

Red Hot Ingredient: Mushrooms

- B-complex vitamins, especially niacin and riboflavin
- Copper, potassium, and selenium
- Fiber

Lentil Stew

Red Hot Mamas around the world enjoy this dish. It's a staple in Blue Zones, where people are known to live the longest. Perhaps the high vitamin, mineral, and amino acid content of its legumes is the answer. And, this dish is delicious, quick, and easy to make. Add a salad for a healthy light meal.

Yield: 4 servings

1 cup lentils, washed and drained

2 large carrots, diced

1 rib celery, diced

1 (8-ounce) can tomato sauce

½ cup canned chickpeas, drained and rinsed

1 teaspoon ground cumin

½ teaspoon ground coriander

½ teaspoon snipped fresh dill

Pour 3 cups of water into a medium-size saucepan and add the lentils. Bring to a boil over high heat and add all the other ingredients. Lower the heat and simmer, covered, stirring occasionally, for about 40 minutes, or until the lentils are tender.

—*Dr. Mache's Kitchen*

Per serving: 215 Cal.; 27 GI; 15 g Prot.; 38 g Carb.; 1 g SFA; 1 g MUFA; 1 g PUFA; 0.1 g Omega-3; 64 mg Calc.; 359 mg Sod.; 848 mg Pot.; 6 mg Iron; 0 mg Phytoestrogen; 11 g Fiber

9

SALADS

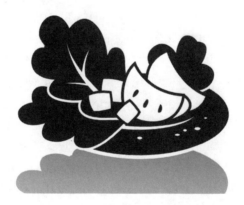

Watermelon and Watercress Salad

This light and healthy salad is great to serve for lunch. To save time, you can make the dressing ahead of time. This is a perfect addition to a summer barbecue or light luncheon. No matter how you slice it, watermelon is great for you, rich in electrolytes, which we lose when we perspire during those hot flashes.

Yield: 4 to 6 servings

Vinaigrette:
2 shallots
½ cup orange juice
½ cup rice wine vinegar
2 teaspoons salt
1½ cups canola oil
¼ cup sesame oil

Salad:
4 bunches watercress
4 cups watermelon, cut into large dice
¼ cup pecans, toasted

Red Hot Ingredient: Watermelon

- Vitamins A, B complex, and E
- Potassium and sodium
- Antioxidants

Power Produce

Use fruits and/or vegetables to replace some of the other foods you're eating to unleash their power and reduce the calories in your diet.

To make the vinaigrette, put the shallots, orange juice, vinegar, and salt in a food processor and puree until smooth. Combine the canola and sesame oils in a mixing bowl and pour in a steady stream into the processor while running. When the vinaigrette is thoroughly blended, pour it into a cruet and refrigerate.

To make the salad, wash the watercress well and remove any large stems. Combine the watercress and watermelon in a mixing bowl and toss with ½ cup of the vinaigrette. (The remaining vinaigrette can be refrigerated and used for another salad.) To serve, arrange the salad pleasingly on serving plates and sprinkle with the toasted pecans.

—*Chef Tres Hundertmark*

Per serving: 482 Cal.; 63 GI; 1 g Prot.; 9 g Carb.; 4 g SFA; 30 g MUFA; 15 g PUFA; 4 g Omega-3; 14 mg Calc.; 605 mg Sod.; 161 mg Pot.; 0.4 mg Iron; 0 mg Phytoestrogen; 1 g Fiber

Dungeness Crab Salad with Peas, Thai Basil, Greens, Mint, and Meyer Lemon Vinaigrette

This delectable salad, made with the freshest of ingredients, is truly refreshing. Dungeness crab is the best crab on earth, and low in fat. Peas contain lutein, which may reduce the risk of cataracts and macular degeneration.

Yield: 4 servings

Lemon Syrup:
1 cup freshly squeezed Meyer lemon juice
1 cup sugar

Lemon Vinaigrette:
½ cup lemon syrup (above)
½ cup grapeseed oil
Juice of 2 Meyer lemons
Rice wine vinegar

Basil Oil:
¾ cup chopped basil
6 tablespoons grapeseed oil
Salt

Salad:
½ pound Dungeness crabmeat
⅓ cup frozen green peas, thawed
1 tablespoon julienned fresh mint
1 tablespoon julienned fresh Thai basil
Salt and pepper
¾ cup mixed micro greens

To make the lemon syrup, put the lemon juice and sugar in a saucepan and bring to a gentle boil over medium-high heat. Cook, uncovered, until the syrup has reduced by half. (You will have more lemon syrup than you need for this recipe.)

To make the lemon vinaigrette, you will need to balance it by taste because the acidity of the lemons will vary the amount of lemon juice and vinegar you will need. Combine the lemon syrup, oil, and lemon juice in a mixing bowl. Add the vinegar to taste and balance with more oil if necessary. Set aside.

To make the basil oil, blanch the basil in boiling salted water for 20 seconds and then shock it in ice water. Wring out the water and place in a food processor. Add the oil and puree. Add a touch of salt and put the puree in a stainless-steel saucepan. Bring to a boil over medium-high heat. Turn off the heat, cover, and allow to steep for 15 minutes. Strain the oil through cheesecloth or a chinois strainer. Put the strained oil into a squirt bottle and set aside.

Continues ...

Dungeness Crab Salad . . . (continued)

To make the salad, in a mixing bowl, combine
the crabmeat, peas, mint, and basil and season to taste with the vinaigrette.

Season with salt and pepper and place in a ring
mold. Pack down and remove the ring. Garnish with the micro greens. Serve with the
lemon vinaigrette and basil oil on the side.

—Chef Neal Fraser

> **Red Hot Ingredient:
> Peas**
>
> • Vitamin C
> • Iron
> • Protein
> • Fiber
> • Lutein (a carotenoid)

Per serving: 765 Cal.; 59 GI; 13 g Prot.; 73 g Carb.; 5 g SFA; 8 g
MUFA; 34 g PUFA; 0.4 g Omega-3; 126 mg Calc.; 475 mg Sod.;
440 mg Pot.; 2 mg Iron; 0 mg Phytoestrogen; 2 g Fiber

Asian Tuna Salad

This is a delicious tuna salad with an Asian twist. A must-try! Tuna is loaded with omega-3 fatty acids, which may help reduce the risk of cardiovascular disease. Omega-3s are also beneficial to our skin and may even help reduce risk of some cancers and arthritis.

Yield: 2 servings

Marinade:

3 tablespoons low-sodium soy sauce

½ teaspoon wasabi paste

1 tablespoon sake

1 (7-ounce) piece fresh tuna

Dressing:

4 tablespoons low-sodium soy sauce

2 tablespoons freshly squeezed lime juice

3 teaspoons sesame oil

2 teaspoons brown sugar

Salad:

1 tablespoon sesame oil

1 cup torn field greens

4 grape tomatoes, halved

¼ cucumber, peeled and sliced

To make the marinade, combine the soy sauce, wasabi paste, and sake in a mixing bowl and mix well.

Place the tuna in a shallow dish and cover with the marinade. Cover and place in the refrigerator and marinate for 4 hours.

Meanwhile, to make the dressing, whisk together the soy sauce, lime juice, oil, and brown sugar and set aside.

To make the salad, heat the oil in a small skillet over high heat and sear each side of the tuna (no more than 20 seconds on each side). Arrange the greens, tomatoes, and cucumber on a salad plate and break up the seared tuna and arrange on top of the salad. Drizzle with the dressing and serve.

—Chef Jeffrey S. Merry

Per serving: 334 Cal.; 52 GI; 27 g Prot.; 13 g Carb.; 3 g SFA; 7 g MUFA; 7 g PUFA; 1 g Omega-3; 45 mg Calc.; 1,908 mg Sod.; 493 mg Pot.; 2 mg Iron; 1 mg Phytoestrogen; 1 g Fiber

Summer Salad

The complementary ingredients in this salad will surely soothe your taste buds. Add some grilled or Cajun chicken, and it will be awesome! Field greens are good sources of antioxidants, which may reduce risks of cancer, heart disease, and cataracts. This is a winning recipe to optimize our health.

Yield: 4 servings

6 large handfuls torn mixed field greens

¼ cup walnuts or almonds, candied and/or roasted

¼ cup sun-dried cranberries

4 ounces mozzarella cheese, diced

1 Granny Smith apple, cored and sliced

8 to 10 strawberries, sliced

¼ cup raspberry vinaigrette

Salt and pepper

1 small lemon, quartered

Combine the greens, nuts, cranberries, cheese, apple, and strawberries in a mixing bowl. Add the raspberry vinaigrette and salt and pepper to taste and toss. Serve on four individual plates with a wedge of lemon for each diner. Enjoy!

—John Liberatore

Per serving: 420 Cal.; 50 GI; 14 g Prot.; 32 g Carb.; 6 g SFA; 9 g MUFA; 12 g PUFA; 2 g Omega-3; 291 mg Calc.; 217 mg Sod.; 452 mg Pot.; 2 mg Iron; 0 mg Phytoestrogen; 6 g Fiber

Red Hot Ingredient: Field Greens

• Vitamin C and folic acid
• Fiber
• Antioxidants

Arugula and Tomato Salad

A cousin of broccoli and cauliflower, arugula is a spicy little leaf with a peppery taste that's very popular in Italy. This recipe is low in calories but high in vitamins. Cruciferous vegetables are rich in phytonutrients that may reduce the risk of breast, stomach, and colon cancer.

Yield: 4 servings

⅓ cup extra-virgin olive oil

4 tablespoons freshly squeezed lemon juice

1 tablespoon lemon zest

1 clove garlic, minced

¾ teaspoon sugar

Salt and pepper

8 cups arugula, washed and dried

1 tomato, cut into thin wedges

In a small bowl, combine the oil, lemon juice, lemon zest, garlic, sugar, and salt and pepper to taste and whisk until blended. Set aside.

Place the arugula in a salad bowl and toss with the dressing. Arrange the tomato wedges on top and serve immediately.

—Karen's Cucina

Per serving: 181 Cal.; 48 GI; 1 g Prot.; 4 g Carb.; 2 g SFA; 13 g MUFA; 2 g PUFA; 0.2 g Omega-3; 72 mg Calc.; 16 mg Sod.; 242 mg Pot.; 1 mg Iron; 0 mg Phytoestrogen; 1 g Fiber

Red Hot Ingredient: Arugula

- Vitamins A, B₂, and C, and folic acid
- Calcium, copper, iron, magnesium, manganese, potassium, and zinc

Spinach Salad with Feta and Prosciutto

You will receive great raves after serving this salad. Spinach has a winning combination of vitamins, fiber, and antioxidants—useful for fighting and preventing a number of diseases, including cancer, and may also preserve eye health and aid in prevention of heart disease and cancer.

Popeye loves this salad!

Yield: 4 servings

¾ pound baby spinach, washed and dried

¼ cup extra-virgin olive oil

1 clove garlic, diced

¼ cup toasted pine nuts

¼ cup diced prosciutto

Salt and pepper

½ cup crumbled feta cheese

Red Hot Ingredient: Spinach

• Vitamin s A, B$_6$, E, and K, and folic acid

• Calcium, iron, and magnesium

• Omega-3 fatty acids

• Antioxidants

Place the spinach in a salad bowl. In a small skillet, heat the olive oil over medium-high heat. Add the garlic and sauté for about 3 minutes, until golden brown. Lower the heat to low and add the pine nuts, prosciutto, and salt and pepper to taste and cook for an additional 5 minutes. Add to the spinach with the feta cheese and toss. Serve immediately.

—*Karen's Cucina*

Per serving: 261 Cal.; 37 GI; 8 g Prot.; 5 g Carb.; 5 g SFA; 12 g MUFA; 4 g PUFA; 0.3 g Omega-3; 180 mg Calc.; 403 mg Sod.; 574 mg Pot.; 3 mg Iron; 0 mg Phytoestrogen; 2 g Fiber

Tuna and Bean Salad

You'll get lots of requests for this recipe. It's got the great fiber, B vitamins, and iron benefits of the cannellini beans, and its combination of tuna and vegetables is delicious.

Yield: 4 servings

2 (7-ounce) cans Italian tuna

2 cups canned cannellini beans, drained and rinsed

¼ cup red onion, diced

6 tablespoons capers, drained

½ cup celery, diced

1 Roma tomato, diced

3 tablespoons freshly squeezed lemon juice

6 tablespoons extra-virgin olive oil

Salt and pepper

Combine the tuna, beans, onions, capers, celery, and tomato in a large bowl. Whisk together the lemon juice, olive oil, and salt and pepper to taste and toss with the tuna mixture. Serve immediately.

—*Karen's Cucina*

Per serving: 147 Cal.; 51 GI; 26 g Prot.; 7 g Carb.; 0.2 g SFA; 0.1 g MUFA; 0.4 g PUFA; 0.3 g Omega-3; 48 mg Calc.; 933 mg Sod.; 420 mg Pot.; 2.5 mg Iron; 0 mg Phytoestrogen; 3 g Fiber

Red Hot Ingredient: Tuna

- Vitamin D
- Protein
- Omega-3 fatty acids

Watercress Salad with Fennel

This recipe is rich in phytonutrients and fiber. It is very different, very fresh, and very good! Watercress, which contains vitamins A and C, calcium, and iron, may help as a diuretic and aid digestion.

Yield: 4 servings

2 large heads fennel

1 bunch watercress

¼ cup extra-virgin olive oil

1 tablespoon white wine vinegar

2 tablespoons capers, drained

¼ teaspoon sugar

Salt and pepper

Red Hot Ingredient: Fennel

- Vitamin C and folic acid
- Calcium, iron, magnesium, manganese, phosphorus, and potassium
- Fiber

Wash, dry, and trim the fennel, removing any blemished leaves. Cut each head of fennel in half, slice as thinly as possible, and place in a large salad bowl.

Rinse and dry the watercress and cut off any tough stems. Add to the salad bowl with the fennel.

In a small bowl, combine the olive oil, vinegar, capers, sugar, and salt and pepper to taste and mix well. Pour over the fennel and watercress and toss lightly. Serve immediately.

—Karen's Cucina

Per serving: 158 Cal.; 67 GI; 1.5 g Prot.; 9 g Carb.; 2 g SFA; 10 g MUFA; 2 g PUFA; 0.1 g Omega-3; 60 mg Calc.; 189 mg Sod.; 490 mg Pot.; 1 mg Iron; 0 mg Phytoestrogen; 4 g Fiber

Tortellini and Olive Salad

This tortellini salad is good, quick, and easy to make. It's a hit at luncheons and potluck dinners, and can be served either cold or hot. The vitamin C in the tomatoes is a recognized antioxidant that may help protect cells from the risk of cancer, diabetes, and heart and lung disease.

Yield: 4 servings

¾ pound tortellini pasta

½ cup chopped spinach

½ cup sliced pitted black olives

½ cup sun-dried tomatoes, diced

¼ cup freshly grated Parmesan cheese

Juice of 1 lemon

¼ cup extra-virgin olive oil

3 cloves garlic, minced

Salt and pepper

Cook the pasta al dente, according to the package instructions. Drain and transfer to a salad bowl. Add the spinach, olives, sun-dried tomatoes, and Parmesan cheese to the pasta. In a small bowl, whisk together the lemon juice, olive oil, and garlic and toss with the pasta mixture. Season with salt and pepper to taste and serve immediately.

—*Karen's Cucina*

Per serving: 372 Cal.; 62 GI; 13 g Prot.; 23 g Carb.; 7 g SFA; 14 g MUFA; 2 g PUFA; 0.2 g Omega-3; 268 mg Calc.; 576 mg Sod.; 353 mg Pot.; 3 mg Iron; 0 mg Phytoestrogen; 2 g Fiber

Roasted Beet and Asparagus Salad

This recipe is a wonderful way to blend together the health benefits of beets and asparagus. Beets contain potent antioxidants and nutrients; they may also lower blood pressure and help prevent cardiovascular disease. Asparagus, a member of the lily family that also includes leeks, garlic and onions, has a calcium-to-magnesium ratio of 2:1, which is just the way your body likes it. Spruce up any meal, including holiday meals, with this unique salad.

Yield: 4 servings

5 small beets, washed and trimmed
1 pound thin asparagus, ends trimmed
¾ cup extra-virgin olive oil
¼ cup balsamic vinegar
Salt and pepper
8 cups torn lettuce

Red Hot Ingredient: Asparagus

• Vitamins A, C, and K, and folic acid
• Calcium and magnesium

Let Off Some Steam!
Steamed vegetables are delicious and low in calories. Steam until the color is bright and try not to overcook them.

Preheat the oven to 400°F.

Wrap the beets in aluminum foil and place on a rack in the oven. Roast for 1 hour, or until they can easily be pierced with a knife. Remove from the oven and let cool. When cool, peel and slice and set aside.

Steam the asparagus for about 5 minutes, until tender, and then plunge into ice cold water to stop the cooking. Drain and set aside.

In a small bowl, whisk together the oil, vinegar, and salt and pepper to taste. Place the lettuce on a serving platter and arrange the asparagus spears and beets on top. Pour the dressing over the top and serve immediately.

—*Karen's Cucina*

Per serving: 450 Cal.; 59 GI; 5 g Prot.; 18 g Carb.; 5 g SFA; 29 g MUFA; 4 g PUFA; 0.3 g Omega-3; 74 mg Calc.; 107 mg Sod.; 720 mg Pot.; 4 mg Iron; 0.06 mg Phytoestrogen; 6 g Fiber

Caprese Salad

This is a colorful, refreshing, and delicious salad that is especially good on very hot days. Serve with some crusty bread and extra-virgin olive oil for dipping. While simple, the cheese and tomatoes' vitamins and minerals work overtime to promote healthy skin and vision and the formation red blood cells, as well as to lower cholesterol and blood pressure and possibly reduce our risk of heart disease.

Yield: 4 servings

2 medium-size vine-ripe tomatoes, sliced

7 ounces part-skim, low-sodium mozzarella, sliced thinly

5 tablespoons chopped fresh basil

2 tablespoons extra-virgin olive oil

1 tablespoon lemon juice

Salt and pepper

On a serving platter, arrange the tomatoes and cheese in overlapping rows and sprinkle the basil over the top.

Whisk together the olive oil, lemon juice, and salt and pepper to taste and drizzle over the tomatoes and cheese and serve immediately.

—*Karen's Cucina*

Per serving: 285 Cal.; 40 GI; 16 g Prot.; 5 g Carb.; 7 g SFA; 7 g MUFA; 1 g PUFA; 0.1 g Omega-3; 524 mg Calc.; 377 mg Sod.; 213 mg Pot.; 0.3 mg Iron; 0 mg Phytoestrogen; 1 g Fiber

Red Hot Ingredient: Mozzarella Cheese

• Vitamins A, B_2, B_6, D, and E

Salade Niçoise

This fabulous salad celebrates the veggies of the season and pairs them with tuna. Talk about good food that's good for you! Tuna is a great source of omega-3 fatty acids. Combine that with green beans, potatoes, lettuce, and tomatoes, which are packed with nutrients, and it's a winning combination.

Yield: 4 servings

Dressing:
2 tablespoons freshly squeezed lemon juice
Pinch of sugar
2 teaspoons anchovy paste
1 teaspoon Dijon mustard
2 tablespoons minced shallots
Pinch of pepper
¼ cup extra-virgin olive oil

Salad:
4 small new potatoes, unpeeled
½ pound green beans, trimmed
1 head tender baby lettuce, leaves separated
1 (7-ounce) can solid white tuna, drained and flaked
2 hard-boiled eggs, quartered lengthwise
¾ cup Niçoise olives, pitted
15 cherry tomatoes
1 pound tomatoes, cut into ¼-inch slices

To make the dressing, in a small bowl combine the lemon juice, sugar, anchovy paste, mustard, shallots, and pepper. Slowly whisk in the olive oil.

Put the potatoes in a small saucepan and cover with water. Bring to a boil over high heat. Once boiling, lower the heat and simmer until the potatoes are tender, about 10 minutes. Drain, halve, and set aside.

Fill a saucepan with 2 inches of water and bring to a boil over high heat. Add the beans and bring to a boil again. Lower the heat and simmer for about 8 minutes, just until they are tender. Drain and set aside.

Place the lettuce leaves in a serving bowl and drizzle with half the dressing. Arrange the tuna, eggs, olives, potatoes, cherry tomatoes, and tomato slices decoratively over the lettuce. Drizzle with the remaining dressing and serve immediately.

—*Karen's Cucina*

Per serving: 316 Cal.; 48 GI; 18 g Prot.; 16 g Carb.; 3.5 g SFA; 14 g MUFA; 3 g PUFA; 0.3 g Omega-3; 99 mg Calc.; 1,004 mg Sod.; 818 mg Pot.; 3 mg Iron; 0 mg Phytoestrogen; 5.5 g Fiber

Celery and Walnut Salad

Enjoy the great mix of sweet and crunchy ingredients in this simple and surprisingly delicious salad! Walnuts have been linked to protection against coronary heart disease. Mineral-rich celery is also a good source of vitamin C, which helps supports our immune system.

Yield: 4 servings

6 ribs celery, cut into ⅛-inch slices

1 cup walnuts, toasted

20 pitted black olives

2 ounces Parmigiano-Reggiano cheese, cut into ¼-inch pieces

6 tablespoons extra-virgin olive oil

1 tablespoon red wine vinegar

½ teaspoon dried oregano

Salt and pepper

Combine the celery, walnuts, olives, and cheese in a salad bowl. In a small bowl, whisk together the olive oil, vinegar, and oregano and toss with the celery mixture, adding salt and pepper to taste. Serve immediately.

—*Karen's Cucina*

Per serving: 433 Cal.; 32 GI; 9 g Prot.; 7 g Carb.; 6 g SFA; 19 g MUFA; 14 g PUFA; 2.5 g Omega-3; 238 mg Calc.; 451 mg Sod.; 289 mg Pot.; 2 mg Iron; 0 mg Phytoestrogen; 3 g Fiber

Red Hot Ingredient: Walnuts

• Vitamins B$_2$ and E, and folic acid

• Calcium, copper, magnesium, manganese, and zinc

• Omega-3 fatty acids

Roasted Beet Salad with Grapefruit and Chive Vinaigrette

This unique combination of delicious ingredients gives this salad a fantastic flavor. Use locally grown heirloom beets when available. Grapefruit is high in insoluble fiber, which helps combat constipation, and is a great source of vitamin C.

Yield: 4 servings

Vinaigrette:

1 egg (Note: Using a raw egg does carry a slight risk of salmonella.)

¼ cup white wine vinegar

½ cup chopped chives

¼ cup flaxseed oil

½ cup canola oil

Salt

Salad:

1 pound beets, trimmed

¼ cup olive oil

Salt

4 cups (½ pound) organic mixed greens (spinach or arugula will also work)

2 large grapefruits, segmented

1 head fennel, shaved or sliced very thinly

Salt and pepper

To make the vinaigrette, put the egg, vinegar, and chives in a food processor and blend until well mixed. Combine the oils, and then slowly add them to the food processor. Blend until the mixture begins to emulsify and turn pale green. If the mixture gets too thick, add up to ¼ cup of water. Season with salt to taste and set aside.

To make the salad, preheat the oven to 400°F. Lightly toss the beets in the olive oil and salt to taste and place on a baking sheet. Cover with foil and bake for 1 hour, or until tender. Let cool and then peel and cut the beets into a large dice.

On a large plate, arrange the mixed greens, beets, grapefruit segments, and fennel. Finish with the chive vinaigrette and season with salt and pepper to taste. Serve immediately.

—*Donnie Ferneau Jr., CEC*

Per serving: 638 Cal.; 43 GI; 6 g Prot.; 31 g Carb.; 5 g SFA; 30 g MUFA; 18 g PUFA; 10 g Omega-3; 108 mg Calc.; 155 mg Sod.; 1,063 mg Pot.; 2 mg Iron; 0.1 mg Phytoestrogen; 8 g Fiber

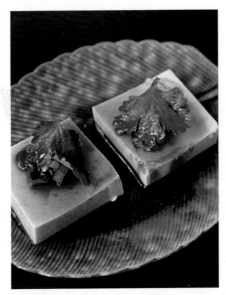

Cold Tofu with Cilantro, Green Onions,
and Soy Sesame Sauce, page 180

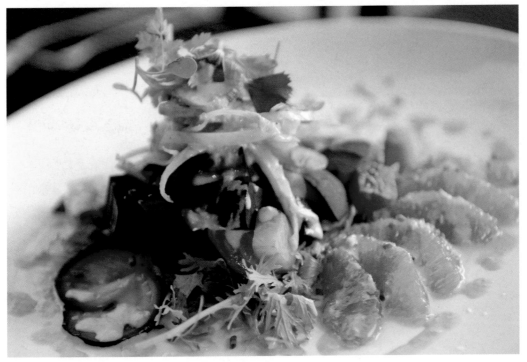

Roasted Beet Salad with Grapefruit and Chive Vinaigrette, page 110

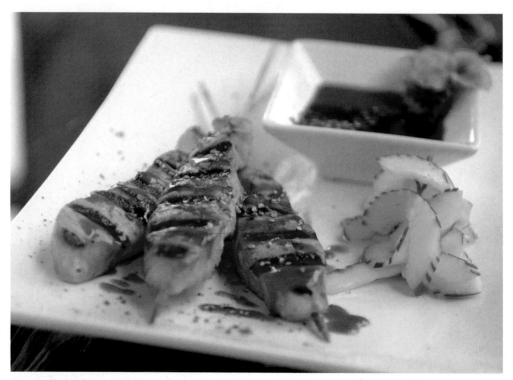

Soy-Grilled Salmon Skewers, page 150

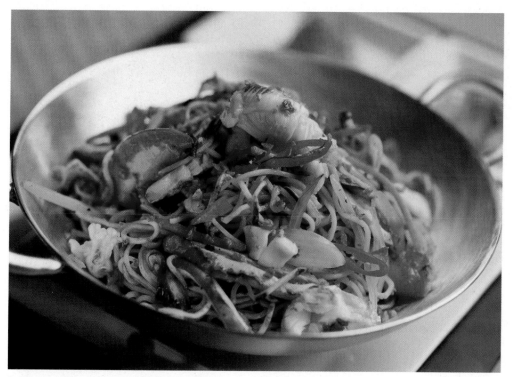
Lobster and Duck Chow Mein, page 161

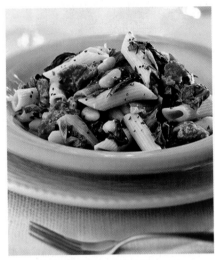

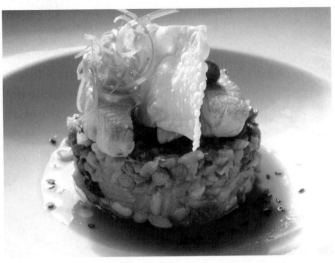

Tuscan-Style Penne with White Beans
and Grilled Chicken and Basil, page 121

Pan-Seared Sardines, Slow-Cooked Grains, Swiss Chard,
Golden Raisins, Pine Nuts, and Smoked Paprika, page 66

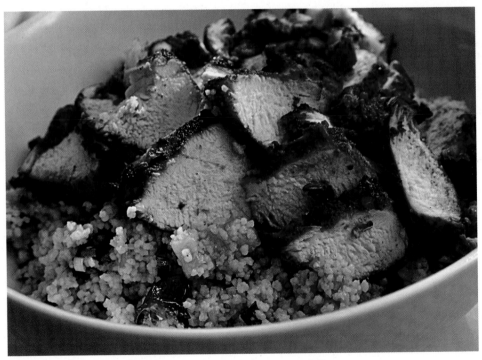

Moroccan Chicken over Apricot-Cranberry Couscous, page 166

Shepherd's Salad

This salad evolved as a celebration of the incredible spring greens received from Your Kitchen Garden Farm in Canby, Oregon, and it appears on the menu at Nostrana in Portland every spring. Its vivid colors are best showcased on a white platter or white serving plates. This salad is a great source of calcium, magnesium, iron, and vitamins A, C, E, and folic acid.

Yield: 4 servings

Pickled Red Onions:
2 medium-size red onions
½ cup apple cider vinegar
1½ tablespoons sugar
3 tablespoons olive oil
1½ teaspoons salt
Generous pinch of pepper

Salad:
6 cups assorted greens, varying in color, texture, and taste (The restaurant uses mizuna, arugula, rustic arugula, mâche, and chrysanthemum leaf)
1 farm-fresh egg
1 large shallot, minced
2 tablespoons sherry vinegar
Salt
6 to 8 tablespoons walnut oil
½ cup creamy, fresh goat cheese
4 slices rustic bread, preferably ciabatta
Walnuts, as local as possible, or, if not, toasted lightly
½ cup pickled red onions (above)
Fleur de Sel sea salt (or Maldon sea salt) (The restaurant uses Flor de Sal, Portuguese sea salt)
Freshly ground pepper

To make the pickled red onions, peel the onions, leaving the stem ends intact; cut into sixths (or eighths, if large). In a medium-size non-reactive saucepan, combine ½ cup of water, and the onion, vinegar, sugar, olive oil, salt, and pepper. Bring to a boil and cook, stirring often, for 5 minutes. Remove from the heat and let the onions cool in the liquid.

To make the salad, wash the greens, dry well, and chill.

Hard-boil the egg (see Tip). Set aside.

Squeeze the shallots in a clean kitchen towel to remove any bitter juices. Place in a small mixing bowl. Add the vinegar and salt to taste. Stir well and let sit for 30 minutes (the shallot will soften in bitterness).

Slowly whisk the walnut oil into the vinegar mixture to emulsify, and then season with salt and pepper to taste.

Preheat the oven or toaster oven broiler.

Continues ...

Shepherd's Salad (continued)

Lightly spread about 2 tablespoons of the goat cheese over each of the ciabatta slices and place under the broiler until golden.

Toss the greens and the walnuts together with enough dressing to coat well, but do not drown them. Arrange on a white platter or on individual plates. Top with the pickled onion and egg quarters, sprinkle with sea salt and a few grindings of pepper, and serve immediately with the bread and cheese.

—*Chef Cathy Whims*

Per serving: 432 Cal.; 60 GI; 12 g Prot.; 43 g Carb.; 4 g SFA; 5 g MUFA; 13 g PUFA; 2 g Omega-3; 91 mg Calc.; 1,272 mg Sod.; 346 mg Pot.; 4 mg Iron; 0 mg Phytoestrogen; 3 g Fiber

Tip:

To hard-boil the egg, first, use a farm-fresh egg. Place the egg in a saucepan and cover with cold water. Bring to a boil, and then immediately remove from the heat and cover the saucepan. Set a timer for 7 minutes. When the timer sounds, immediately drain the egg and run cold water over it until it is cool. Peel and quarter lengthwise.

Canlis Salad

This salad has been on the Canlis menu in Seattle, in a myriad of versions since 1950. Executive Chef Jason Franey's preparation incorporates the same ingredients as the original, whose combined nutrients may help to improve heart health, prevent strokes, lower cholesterol and blood pressure levels, and even help fight certain cancers, as well as protect against heart and degenerative eye diseases.

Yield: 1 serving

Seasoned Croutons (Makes about 4 cups to serve 8):

¼ cup butter (½ stick)

1 tablespoon salt

1 tablespoon dried oregano

1 tablespoon Italian seasoning

1 teaspoon freshly ground pepper

1 teaspoon garlic powder

4 cups European-style white bread, cut into ¼-inch cubes

Dressing (Makes about 1 cup to serve 8):

1 coddled egg (see Tip)

¼ cup freshly squeezed lemon juice

1 teaspoon freshly ground pepper

½ cup olive oil

Salad (per serving):

¼ head romaine lettuce, washed and cut into 1-inch pieces

Heirloom cherry tomatoes, halved or quartered

½ cup croutons (above)

2 tablespoons chopped green onion

2 tablespoons well-done chopped bacon, drained

1 teaspoon dried oregano

3 tablespoons freshly grated Romano cheese

2 tablespoons (or to taste) finely chopped fresh mint

Kosher salt and freshly ground pepper

Per serving (salad): 170 Cal.; 47 GI; 12 g Prot.; 10 g Carb.; 5 g SFA; 3 g MUFA; 1 g PUFA; 0.3 g Omega-3; 316 mg Calc.; 457 mg Sod.; 640 mg Pot.; 3 mg Iron; 0 mg Phytoestrogen; 5 g Fiber

Per serving (dressing): 132 Cal.; 33 GI; 1 g Prot.; 1 g Carb.; 2 g SFA; 10 g MUFA; 1 g PUFA; 0.1 g Omega-3; 6 mg Calc.; 9 mg Sod.; 22 mg Pot.; 0 mg Iron; 0 mg Phytoestrogen; 0 g Fiber

Per serving (croutons): 105 Cal.; 60 GI; 2 g Prot.; 10 g Carb.; 3 g SFA; 1 g MUFA; 0.3 g PUFA; 0.05 g Omega-3; 291 mg Calc.; 450 mg Sod.; 44 mg Pot.; 1 mg Iron; 0 mg Phytoestrogen; 1 g Fiber

Continues . . .

Canlis Salad (continued)

To make the croutons, preheat the oven to 300°F. Melt the butter over medium heat in a small skillet. Add the salt, oregano, Italian seasoning, pepper, and garlic powder.

Place the bread cubes in a baking dish, add the melted butter mixture, and toss to mix well. Bake, stirring every 5 minutes, for 30 to 40 minutes, or until crisp and golden brown. Cool completely at room temperature before serving or storing. (Extra croutons keep in an airtight container at room temperature for several days.)

To make the dressing, in a small bowl, beat the egg with the lemon juice and pepper. Still beating, stream in the olive oil and continue beating for a few seconds to create a smooth dressing. Set aside.

To make the salad, in a large, well-seasoned wooden salad bowl, combine the lettuce, tomatoes, ½ cup of the croutons, the green onion, bacon, oregano, half the cheese, half the mint, and a generous sprinkling of kosher salt and freshly ground pepper. Toss the salad dry to distribute the ingredients evenly, then pour on 2 tablespoons of the dressing and toss again.

Transfer the salad to a serving plate. Finish with the remaining cheese and mint and a generous grinding of pepper.

—Chef Jason Franey

Tip:

To coddle an egg, you must make sure the egg is very fresh. Run the egg under warm water until the egg is at room temperature. Place the egg in the shell in a small bowl and then pour boiling water over the egg until it is fully covered. Let the egg sit in the boiling water for 1 minute, then run under very cold water.

Kale with Tofu

The key to this recipe is using fresh kale chopped finely so it cooks in less time. This is a delicious and fast way to include a nutritious green leafy vegetable, rich in calcium and vitamins, along with the benefits of soy. It's a great choice for women with hot flashes and who want to maintain healthy bones.

Yield: 4 servings

2 tablespoons olive oil

3 cups finely chopped kale

½ pound organic firm tofu, cubed

2 to 3 cloves of garlic, chopped finely

Salt and other seasonings, such as garlic, ginger, and freshly ground black pepper

Heat the olive oil in a skillet over medium-high heat. Add the kale, tofu, and garlic and sauté until the kale is deep green and tender. Remove from the heat and season to taste with salt and your choice of other seasonings. Serve over pasta, brown rice, or alone.

—*Hari Kaur Khalsa*

Per serving: 193 Cal.; 44 GI; 7 g Prot.; 6 g Carb.; 1 g SFA; 7 g MUFA; 1 g PUFA; 0.1 g Omega-3; 171 mg Calc.; 27 mg Sod.; 307 mg Pot.; 2 mg Iron; 13 mg Phytoestrogen; 1 g Fiber

Yogi No-Egg Egg Salad

Tofu is the great masquerader, and can taste like egg salad without the cholesterol. It's quick and easy to make. Like all soy dishes, it is a great source of phytoestrogens, calcium, and protein, all of which are essential for women in perimenopause and menopause.

Yield: 4 servings

1 pound firm low-fat tofu

1 large rib celery, chopped

¼ cup finely chopped onion

¼ cup tofu mayonnaise (available in health food stores)

1 tablespoon prepared mustard

Mash the tofu with a fork in a large bowl until it becomes crumbly. Add the celery, onion, mayonnaise, and mustard; mix thoroughly. Serve on whole-grain or pita bread with sliced tomatoes and sprouts.

—Hari Kaur Khalsa

Per serving: 126 Cal.; 44 GI; 10 g Prot.; 4.5 g Carb.; 1 g SFA; 2 g MUFA; 4 g PUFA; 0.3 g Omega-3; 242 mg Calc.; 186 mg Sod.; 249 mg Pot.; 2 mg Iron; 31 mg Phytoestrogen; 2 g Fiber

Yogi Sesame-Yogurt Dressing

When eating raw vegetables, it's great to have a healthy dressing to go with it. According to the yogis, this dressing helps prevent gas, which some people get from eating raw vegetables. This dressing is not only healthy, it's also delicious.

Yield: 3 cups

4 sprigs of fresh parsley, chopped

1 rib celery, chopped

¼ small onion

½ cup sesame seeds

1 clove garlic, sliced

1 cup plain yogurt

½ cup raw sesame oil

2 tablespoons freshly squeezed lemon juice

2 tablespoons soy sauce

1 tablespoon balsamic vinegar

1 teaspoon honey

¼ teaspoon salt

¼ teaspoon pepper

Blend all the ingredients in a food processor on low speed until smooth and serve with a selection of raw vegetables.

—*Hari Kaur Khalsa*

Per serving: 74 Cal.; 49 GI; 2 g Prot.; 3 g Carb.; 1 g SFA; 2 g MUFA; 2 g PUFA; 0.02 g Omega-3; 34 mg Calc.; 165 mg Sod.; 71 mg Pot.; 0.3 mg Iron; 0.05 mg Phytoestrogen; 1 g Fiber

10

PASTAS

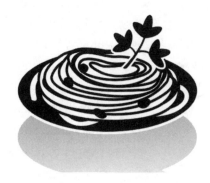

Spaghetti Puttanesca

This is a quick and easy meal to make that is jam-packed with flavors. In Italy, the word puttanesca *has a naughty hidden meaning; there's nothing naughty here, though—this recipe's ingredients may help prevent cancer and promote cardiovascular health. Don't leave out the capers, which contain phytonutrients and antioxidants.*

Yield: 4 servings

¾ pound spaghetti

8 tablespoons extra-virgin olive oil

4 cloves garlic, chopped

1 (4-ounce) can anchovies

Pinch of red pepper flakes

1 (28-ounce) can diced Italian plum tomatoes

50 pitted Italian black olives

5 tablespoons capers, drained and rinsed

Handful of chopped fresh Italian (flat-leaf) parsley

Salt and pepper

Cook the spaghetti al dente according to the package instructions. (I prefer the Barilla brand.) Drain and set aside.

Heat the olive oil in a large skillet over medium heat, and then add the garlic, anchovies, and red pepper flakes and sauté for 3 to 4 minutes. Add the tomatoes and cook for 10 minutes longer, and then add the olives and capers and cook for 5 additional minutes. Add the cooked spaghetti and mix well with the sauce. Stir in the parsley and salt and pepper to taste and serve immediately.

—*Karen's Cucina*

Per serving: 659 Cal.; 43 GI; 18 g Prot.; 76 g Carb.; 5 g SFA; 24 g MUFA; 4 g PUFA; 0.5 g Omega-3; 178 mg Calc.; 1,460 mg Sod.; 566 mg Pot.; 7 mg Iron; 0 mg Phytoestrogen; 10 g Fiber

Tuscan-Style Penne with White Beans and Grilled Chicken and Basil

This pasta dish is an excellent dinner choice. Made with fresh escarole and cooked in broth with sautéed garlic and seasoned chicken, it is super-tasty! Escarole is packed with antioxidants that are essential for optimum health and cancer prevention.

Yield: 4 servings

8 ounces penne rigate pasta

1 tablespoon olive oil

1 teaspoon chopped garlic

2½ cups coarsely chopped escarole

½ cup canned white cannellini beans, drained

4 ounces grilled chicken breast, cut into bite-size pieces

½ cup chicken broth

1 teaspoon chopped fresh basil

Cook the penne pasta al dente according to the package instructions. Drain and set aside.

Heat the oil in a large skillet over medium heat. Add the garlic and sauté until tender but not browned. Add the escarole, beans, chicken, and chicken broth and bring to a simmer, and then add the cooked pasta and cook until heated through.

Transfer to individual bowls and sprinkle with the basil.

—*Chef Jeffrey S. Merry*

Per serving: 258 Cal.; 42 GI; 18 g Prot.; 43 g Carb.; 0.5 g SFA; 0.6 g MUFA; 0.6 g PUFA; 0 g Omega-3; 53 mg Calc.; 117 mg Sod.; 294 mg Pot.; 2 mg Iron; 0 mg Phytoestrogen; 6 g Fiber

Lemon Fettuccine

This recipe is a show-stopper and can be served at an elaborate meal. The intense lemony flavor with the pasta always makes guests ask for seconds. Lemons are the secret health weapon here, with nutrients that promote immunity and fight infection.

Yield: 4 servings

¾ pound fresh or dried fettuccine pasta

4 tablespoons extra-virgin olive oil

3 cloves garlic, chopped

Pinch of red pepper flakes

Juice and zest of 3 lemons

1 tablespoon unsalted butter

Salt and pepper

4 tablespoons chopped fresh Italian (flat-leaf) parsley

¾ cup freshly grated pecorino-Romano cheese

Cook the fettucine al dente according to the package instructions. Drain and set aside.

Heat the olive oil in a large skillet over medium-low heat. Add the garlic and red pepper flakes and sauté for about 3 minutes, until the garlic is tender but not browned. Add the lemon juice and zest, bring to a boil, and then remove from the heat and add the butter and the salt and pepper to taste. Add the cooked fettuccine and toss well. Stir in the parsley and cheese and serve immediately.

—*Karen's Cucina*

Per serving: 490 Cal.; 40 GI; 12 g Prot.; 51 g Carb.; 6 g SFA; 14 g MUFA; 1 g PUFA; 0.2 g Omega-3; 122 mg Calc.; 101 mg Sod.; 160 mg Pot.; 3 mg Iron; 0.03 mg Phytoestrogen; 3 g Fiber

Red Hot Ingredient: Lemons

- Vitamin C
- Calcium and magnesium
- Bioflavenoids
- Pectin
- Limonene

To Lose or Control Weight . . .

Replace 1 cup of the rice or pasta in your dish with 1 cup of chopped vegetables, such as tomatoes, squash, onions, peppers, or broccoli.

Spaghetti with Tuna

There are an infinite number of tuna sauces. This one is quick and easy to make and is surprisingly tasty. The combination of tuna (which is high in protein and a great source of vitamin D and omega-3 fatty acids) and tomatoes is helpful in maintaining good health. To reduce the amount of salt, simply use fewer anchovies.

Yield: 4 servings

¾ pound spaghetti

¼ cup extra-virgin olive oil

3 cloves garlic, chopped

1 (4-ounce) can anchovies

1 (28-ounce) can Italian plum tomatoes

1 (3-ounce) can tuna in olive oil, drained and flaked

8 pitted olives, halved

5 tablespoons capers, drained and rinsed

Pinch of red pepper flakes

Handful of chopped fresh Italian (flat-leaf) parsley

Salt and pepper

In a large saucepan, cook the spaghetti al dente according to the package instructions. Drain and set aside.

Heat the olive oil in a 12-inch skillet over medium-low heat. Add the garlic and sauté until tender but not browned. Add the anchovies, mashing them with a wooden spoon. Add the tomatoes and stir in the tuna, olives, capers, red pepper flakes, and parsley. Simmer on low heat for 10 minutes. Add the spaghetti, mixing it well with the sauce, and cook for 3 to 4 minutes longer, until it is thoroughly mixed and heated through.

Serve immediately.

—*Karen's Cucina*

Per serving: 532 Cal.; 43 GI; 24 g Prot.; 73 g Carb.; 3 g SFA; 12 g MUFA; 3 g PUFA; 0.4 g Omega-3; 143 mg Calc.; 1,168 mg Sod.; 604 mg Pot.; 6 mg Iron; 0 mg Phytoestrogen; 9 g Fiber

Lemon-Walnut Farfalle

This simple, no-fuss recipe is great. The anchovies and walnuts are a great combination. Parmesan cheese is rich in calcium, protein, and phosphorous, which may even act to protect our tooth enamel. To reduce the amount of salt, simply use fewer anchovies.

Yield: 4 servings

¾ pound farfalle pasta

2 tablespoons extra-virgin olive oil

6 cloves garlic, chopped

1 (4-ounce) can anchovies

1 cup finely chopped walnuts

Zest of 1 large lemon

½ cup freshly grated Parmesan cheese

Handful of chopped fresh Italian (flat-leaf) parsley

Cook the pasta al dente according to the package instructions. When it is almost done, remove 1 cup of the cooking water and set aside. When the pasta is done, drain the rest of the water and set the pasta aside.

Heat the olive oil in large skillet over medium-high heat. Add the garlic and sauté for 2 minutes, until tender but not browned. Lower the heat to low and add the anchovies, walnuts, and lemon zest and cook for 3 minutes. Stir the cup of cooking water into the sauce, and then add the pasta and mix well. Transfer to a warmed serving bowl and serve immediately sprinkled with the cheese and parsley.

—*Karen's Cucina*

Per serving: 707 Cal.; 46 GI; 26 g Prot.; 78 g Carb.; 6 g SFA; 9 g MUFA; 15 g PUFA; 3 g Omega-3; 249 mg Calc.; 643 mg Sod.; 328 mg Pot.; 4 mg Iron; 0 mg Phytoestrogen; 6 g Fiber

Penne with Pine Nuts in Tomato Sauce

When time's tight, this is one of the most delicious, easiest (and fastest) solutions.

Yield: 4 servings

¾ pound penne pasta

½ cup pine nuts

4 tablespoons extra-virgin olive oil

4 cloves garlic, chopped

Pinch of red pepper flakes

Salt

1 (28-ounce) can tomatoes

4 tablespoons chopped fresh Italian (flat-leaf) parsley

Handful of chopped fresh basil

¾ tablespoons unsalted butter

¼ cup freshly grated Parmesan cheese

Red Hot Ingredient: Pine Nuts

- Vitamins B_1, B_2, B_3, and E
- Copper, magnesium, manganese, potassium, and zinc
- Amino acids

In a large saucepan, cook the penne al dente according to the package instructions. When it is almost done, remove ¾ cup of the cooking water and set aside. When the pasta is done, drain and set aside.

In a large skillet, toast the pine nuts over medium heat until golden brown. Add the olive oil, garlic, red pepper flakes, and salt to taste and sauté until the garlic is tender but not browned. Add the tomatoes (mashing them with a wooden spoon), parsley and basil. Bring to a boil, and then lower the heat and simmer for 20 minutes. Stir the reserved cooking water into the sauce, and then add the pasta and toss to mix well. Serve with the Parmesan cheese sprinkled over the top.

—*Karen's Cucina*

Per serving: 612 Cal.; 42 GI; 19 g Prot.; 73 g Carb.; 5 g SFA; 14 g MUFA; 8 g PUFA; 0.2 g Omega-3; 207 mg Calc.; 408 mg Sod.; 642 mg Pot.; 6 mg Iron; 0 mg Phytoestrogen; 9.5 g Fiber

Penne with Golden Raisins, Spinach, and Chickpeas

This is a simple, easy recipe that is always a crowd pleaser. Raisins contain boron, a trace mineral, that provides protection against osteoporosis, and they may have cancer-inhibiting properties.

Yield: 4 servings

¾ pound penne pasta

4 tablespoons extra-virgin olive oil

4 cloves garlic, chopped

1 (19-ounce) can chickpeas, drained and rinsed

12 ounces spinach, washed and dried

½ cup golden raisins

Salt

Pinch of red pepper flakes

¾ cup chicken broth

In a large saucepan, cook the penne al dente according to the package instructions. Drain and set aside.

In a large skillet, heat the olive oil over medium-high heat. Add the garlic and sauté until it is a light golden color. Stir in the chickpeas, spinach, raisins, salt to taste, and the red pepper flakes. Add the chicken broth and simmer over low heat for 20 minutes. Add the pasta and toss to mix well.

Serve immediately.

—*Karen's Cucina*

Per serving: 712 Cal.; 45 GI; 28 g Prot.; 116 g Carb.; 2.5 g SFA; 11 g MUFA; 3 g PUFA; 0.3 g Omega-3; 196 mg Calc.; 332 mg Sod.; 1,150 mg Pot.; 9 mg Iron; 2 mg Phytoestrogen; 17 g Fiber

Red Hot Ingredient: Spinach

• Vitamins A, B_6, E, and K, and folic acid

• Calcium, iron, and magnesium

• Omega-3 fatty acids

• Antioxidants

Red Hot Ingredient: Raisins

• Vitamins B_1, B_2, B_6, and C, and niacin

• Boron, iron, phosphorus, and selenium

• Amino acids

• Antioxidants

Linguine with Seafood

Highly recommended! This is an awesome and delicious dish. The flavor from the seafood really makes this sauce. The fish are rich sources of omega-3 fatty acids, essential for cardiovascular health. Scallops are good sources of potassium and magnesium.

Yield: 4 servings

¾ pound linguine pasta

¼ cup extra-virgin olive oil

25 medium shrimp, peeled and deveined

4 ounces medium-size scallops

Salt and pepper

4 ounces calamari

4 ounces fresh crabmeat, flaked

6 cloves garlic, chopped

¼ cup quartered kalamata olives

¼ cup sun-dried tomatoes packed in olive oil (reserve the oil)

1 (28-ounce) can tomatoes

1 tablespoon unsalted butter

¼ cup chopped fresh basil leaves

¼ cup chopped Italian parsley

Cook the linguine al dente according to the package instructions. Drain and set aside.

Heat the olive oil in a large skillet over low heat. Add the shrimp, scallops, and salt and pepper to taste and cook for 3 minutes. Add the calamari, crabmeat, and garlic and cook for an additional 2 minutes. Then add the olives, sun-dried tomatoes, 2 tablespoons of their reserved oil, and the canned tomatoes and cook for 2 more minutes. Add the linguine and toss to mix well, and then stir in the butter, basil, and salt and pepper to taste.

Sprinkle with the parsley and serve immediately.

—*Karen's Cucina*

Per serving: 688 Cal.; 47 GI; 35 g Prot.; 86 g Carb.; 4 g SFA; 12 g MUFA; 3 g PUFA; 0.6 g Omega-3; 173 mg Calc.; 575 mg Sod.; 897 mg Pot.; 8 mg Iron; 0.008 mg Phytoestrogen; 7 g Fiber

Vermicelli with Clam Sauce

This vermicelli has a quick and easy sauce that could be served with any pasta. Clams, high in iron, are the magic ingredient here (many pre- and perimenopausal women have difficulty getting enough iron in their daily diet, resulting in anemia).

Yield: 4 servings

¾ pound vermicelli pasta

½ cup extra-virgin olive oil

6 cloves garlic, sliced thinly

2 (10-ounce) cans chopped clams, with juice

Pinch of red pepper flakes

Salt and pepper

½ cup sliced olives

Juice of 1 lemon

2 cups dry white wine

1 (28-ounce) can tomatoes

½ cup chopped fresh Italian (flat-leaf) parsley

Cook the pasta al dente according to the package instructions. Drain and set aside.

In a large skillet, heat the olive oil over low heat. Add the garlic, clams and their juice, red pepper flakes, and salt and pepper to taste and cook for 4 minutes. Add the olives, lemon juice, wine, tomatoes (mashing them with a wooden spoon), and parsley and cook for an additional 10 minutes. Add the cooked pasta and toss to mix well. Serve immediately.

—*Karen's Cucina*

Per serving: 871 Cal.; 46 GI; 27 g Prot.; 93 g Carb.; 5 g SFA; 23 g MUFA; 4 g PUFA; 0.4 g Omega-3; 185 mg Calc.; 715 mg Sod.; 908 mg Pot.; 19 mg Iron; 0.032 mg Phytoestrogen; 8 g Fiber

Red Hot Ingredient: Clams

- Copper, iron, manganese, phosphorus, potassium, selenium, and zinc
- Protein
- Omega-3 fatty acids

Farfalle with Tomatoes and Goat Cheese

This is an unforgettable, delicious recipe for Italian pasta served vegetarian style. Your guests will ask for seconds. Goat cheese—low in fat, calories, and cholesterol, and a good source of bone-preserving calcium—has a full rich creamy flavor and has fewer carbohydrates than other cheeses, such as cream cheese. Many people who have lactose intolerance find goat cheese more digestible.

Yield: 4 servings

¾ pound farfalle pasta

4 tablespoons extra-virgin olive oil

8 cloves garlic, sliced thinly

1 (28-ounce) can diced Italian plum tomatoes

½ cup pine nuts

Pinch of red pepper flakes

Salt and pepper

1 cup torn fresh basil

6 ounces soft goat cheese, crumbled

Cook the pasta al dente according to the package instructions. Drain and set aside.

Heat the olive oil in a large skillet over medium heat. Add the garlic, tomatoes, pine nuts, red pepper flakes, and salt and pepper to taste and cook for 10 minutes, stirring frequently. Then add the basil and cook for an additional 4 minutes. Add the pasta and cheese and toss to mix well. Serve immediately.

—Karen's Cucina

Per serving: 686 Cal.; 47 GI; 21 g Prot.; 85 g Carb.; 5 g SFA; 14 g MUFA; 8 g PUFA; 0.2 g Omega-3; 131 mg Calc.; 340 mg Sod.; 640 mg Pot.; 7 mg Iron; 0.032 mg Phytoestrogen; 7 g Fiber

What's in Your Stomach?

Make two fists with your hands and hold them in front of your stomach. This is the total amount of food you should have in your stomach at any one time. The yogic prescription for filling your stomach is one-third food, one-third water, and one-third space for digestion.

Smashed Tomatoes and Penne

This recipe from Good Carbs, Bad Carbs *author Johanna Burani allows 2½ ounces of pasta per person, which is plenty for a light meal or* i primi *(first course). With pasta, take notice of the cooking times the manufacturer suggests, but ignore the suggested serving size. They are almost always too much pasta for a single meal, sometimes suggesting you use an entire pound of pasta for four people! That's serious carb overload for most people.*

Yield: 4 servings

4 tablespoons extra-virgin olive oil

2 large cloves garlic, minced

1 pound grape (cherry) tomatoes, washed and halved lengthwise

1 teaspoon salt

½ pound penne or other short pasta

Fresh basil leaves (optional)

Freshly grated Romano cheese (optional)

Per serving: 388 Cal.; 47 GI; 10 g Prot.; 48 g Carb.; 2 g SFA; 10 g MUFA; 2 g PUFA; 0.1 g Omega-3; 25 mg Calc.; 228 mg Sod.; 344 mg Pot.; 2 mg Iron; 0 mg Phytoestrogen; 4 g Fiber

In a medium-size saucepan, heat 2 tablespoons of the olive oil over medium-low heat for just a minute. Add the garlic and tomatoes and give it all a good stir, then cover the saucepan and let it simmer gently for 10 minutes, stirring occasionally.

Remove the pan from the heat and, with the back of a wooden spoon or a fork, lightly smash the tomatoes.

In the meantime, bring a large saucepan of 2 to 3 quarts of water to the boil, add the salt, and cook the pasta for 10 to 11 minutes, until al dente, following the package instructions. Do not overcook. Drain the pasta and add it to the saucepan with the tomatoes and garlic. Drizzle the remaining olive oil over the pasta mixture, stir so it is all well combined, and serve immediately. Top with fresh basil leaves and freshly grated Romano cheese if you wish.

—*University of Sydney Glycemic Index and GI Database*

Pesto

This is a quick and easy pesto sauce to top any pasta. It makes a great change from red sauce. The compounds found in basil have antioxidant and anticancer properties—and it tastes great!

Yield: 2 cups pesto (eight ¼-cup servings)

2 cups chopped fresh basil

4 cloves garlic, chopped

1 cup pine nuts

1 cup olive oil

¾ cup freshly grated, reduced-fat Parmesan cheese

¼ cup freshly grated Romano cheese

Salt and pepper

Combine the basil, garlic, and nuts in the bowl of a food processor (or use a blender to process half the recipe at a time). Pulse a few times and then pour in the olive oil in a steady stream while the motor is running. Shut the motor off and add the cheeses, a pinch of salt, and a liberal grinding of pepper. Process briefly to combine, then scrape out into a bowl. Serve with your favorite pasta dish or soup. (This sauce can be stored for up to a week in the refrigerator.)

—Cynthia Niles

Per serving: 397 Cal.; 27 GI; 6 g Prot.; 3 g Carb.; 6 g SFA; 24 g MUFA; 9 g PUFA; 0.3 g Omega-3; 172 mg Calc.; 196 mg Sod.; 154 mg Pot.; 2 mg Iron; 0 mg Phytoestrogen; 1 g Fiber

Don't Pass the Cream!

Use nonfat sour cream or skim milk thickened with cornstarch instead of cream in pasta sauces. First dissolve cornstarch in a little cold water, using 1 tablespoon of cornstarch for each 1 cup of liquid you are replacing. You can also use 1 tablespoon of flour whisked into 1 cup of nonfat milk as an alternative to heavy cream.

Tip:

Because this recipe is high in calories, be sure to serve it as a complement to a low-calorie pasta dish.

Pasta with Braised Garden Vegetable Ratatouille

This wonderful low-calorie pasta can be a complete meal with the addition of a salad. You can replace the fresh tomato sauce with 28 ounces of your favorite low-sodium tomato sauce. The zucchini is the magic Red Hot ingredient here, with its numerous health benefits, from helping to build strong bones to keeping our immune system healthy. It may also protect us against developing rheumatoid arthritis and osteoarthritis.

Yield: 4 servings

Tomato Sauce:
3 pounds plum tomatoes, cored
1 tablespoon olive oil
¼ large onion, diced
2 cloves garlic, minced
½ cup finely chopped fresh basil
Salt and pepper

Braised Vegetables:
1 tablespoon olive oil
1 medium-size onion, diced
2 cloves garlic, minced
1 medium-size summer squash, sliced thinly
1 medium-size zucchini, sliced thinly
1 medium-size eggplant, peeled and cubed
3 tablespoons finely chopped fresh basil

Pasta:
6 ounces pasta (long, flat pasta is best, such as fettuccine)
Salt and pepper
½ cup grated Parmesan cheese

To make the sauce, puree the tomatoes in a food processor and set aside.

Heat the olive oil in a 4-quart saucepan over medium heat. Add the onion and sauté for 5 minutes, or until tender and translucent. Add the garlic and sauté for 30 seconds, and then stir in the tomato puree and basil and simmer for 20 minutes over medium heat. Stir in the salt and pepper to taste.

While the tomato sauce is simmering, prepare the braised vegetables.

In a large, heavy saucepan, heat the olive oil over medium heat. Add the onion and sauté until tender and translucent. Add the garlic and sauté for an additional 30 seconds. Add the summer squash, zucchini, and eggplant and stir to combine, adding more oil if needed. Sprinkle with the basil and then stir in the tomato sauce and simmer for 30 minutes over low heat, stirring occasionally.

To make the pasta, cook it according to the package instructions. Drain the pasta and add it to the saucepan with the ratatouille. Toss well and add salt and pepper to taste if necessary. Garnish with the Parmesan cheese and serve immediately.

—*Brad Stevens, Tony Murillo, and Heather Tsatsarones, MS, RD, LDN*

Per serving: 409 Cal.; 47 GI; 17 g Prot.; 60 g Carb.; 4 g SFA; 7 g MUFA; 2 g PUFA; 0.2 g Omega-3; 277 mg Calc.; 437 mg Sod.; 1,628 mg Pot.; 4 mg Iron; 0 mg Phytoestrogen; 13 g Fiber

11

ENTRÉES

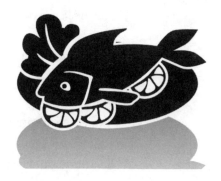

Pan-Roasted Haddock

This is a great recipe with a truly Mediterranean flavor that you can put together in no time.

Yield: 1 serving

1 (½-pound) haddock fillet

2 teaspoons olive oil

⅛ teaspoon freshly ground pepper

½ tablespoon minced shallot

½ cup halved cherry tomatoes

⅛ cup chopped olives

½ tablespoon capers, rinsed and chopped

1 teaspoon dried oregano

½ teaspoon balsamic vinegar

Red Hot Ingredient: Haddock

- Vitamins A, B complex, and D
- Magnesium, phosphorus, selenium, and zinc
- Omega-3 fatty acids

Preheat the oven to 450°F.

Rub the haddock fillet with 1 teaspoon of the olive oil, sprinkle with the pepper, and place in a small roasting pan. Bake for about 15 minutes (the fish should easily flake with a fork).

While the fish is roasting, heat the remaining teaspoon of olive oil in a skillet over medium-high heat. Add the shallot and sauté for about 20 seconds. Add the tomatoes, olives, and capers and sauté for about 30 seconds, and then stir in the oregano and vinegar. Set aside and keep warm.

When the haddock is cooked, place it on a plate, spoon the warm tapenade over it, and serve.

—*Chef Jeffrey S. Merry*

Per serving: 263 Cal.; 51 GI; 44 g Prot.; 9 g Carb.; 1 g SFA; 2 g MUFA; 1 g PUFA; 1 g Omega-3; 93 mg Calc.; 463 mg Sod.; 987 mg Pot.; 2 mg Iron; 0.007 mg Phytoestrogen; 3 g Fiber

Sautéed Trout with Citrus

This flaky, juicy trout dish with a spritz of citrus is vibrant and refreshing. The fruits in this recipe are a good source of fiber and vitamin C, which keeps our immune system strong and may help prevent heart disease and cancer.

Yield: 4 servings

Seasoning:

1½ tablespoons salt

1 teaspoon chili powder

½ teaspoon ground cumin

½ teaspoon ground coriander

Fish:

Cooking spray

4 (6-ounce) sunburst trout fillets

1 ruby red grapefruit section, quartered

2 navel orange sections, halved

2 blood orange sections, halved

4 satsuma sections

½ cup orange marmalade

2 green onions, sliced diagonally

4 sprigs of fresh cilantro

To make the seasoning, combine the salt, chili powder, cumin, and coriander and store in a spice bottle.

Preheat the oven to 400°F. Spray a baking dish with cooking spray.

Season each fish fillet with ¼ teaspoon of the seasoning. Grill or bake the fish for 10 to 12 minutes, or until cooked through.

While the fish is cooking, divide the citrus sections equally among four small bowls and combine each with 2 tablespoons of the marmalade.

To serve, place a fillet of fish on individual serving plates and top each with the citrus sections mixture, green onions, and a sprig of cilantro.

—*Chef Tres Hundertmark*

Per serving: 489 Cal.; 44 GI; 38 g Prot.; 60 g Carb.; 2 g SFA; 6 g MUFA; 3 g PUFA; 2 g Omega-3; 180 mg Calc.; 2,980 mg Sod.; 1,133 mg Pot.; 3 mg Iron; 0.115 mg Phytoestrogen; 6 g Fiber

Olive Oil–Poached Halibut with Black Chickpea Tapenade

This fish dish has a tasty and elegant pairing of ingredients and makes a beautiful presentation. Chickpeas contain the amino acid tryptophan, which may helps us get a good night's sleep. Use reduced-sodium chicken broth to lower the sodium content of this recipe.

Yield: 6 servings

Chickpea Tapenade:

2½ cups black or regular chickpeas (soaked overnight)

4 quarts chicken or vegetable broth

1 onion, halved

1 carrot

1 clove garlic

1 (2-ounce) piece of pork (prosciutto, bacon, ham hock) (optional)

3 tablespoons olive oil

2 ripe tomatoes, diced

1 red bell pepper, roasted, seeded, peeled, and diced

12 black olives, chopped

Zest of 2 lemons

6 tablespoons white balsamic vinegar

4 shallots, chopped

1 bunch of fresh parsley, chopped

Salt and pepper

Fish:

4 quarts olive oil

6 (6-ounce) thick pieces halibut

To make the chickpea tapenade, put the chickpeas in a large heavy saucepan. Add the broth, onion, carrot, garlic, and pork (if using). Bring to a boil and then lower the heat and simmer, covered, for 1 to 2 hours, until the beans are tender. Drain and put the chickpeas in a large bowl. Discard the onion, carrot, garlic, and pork.

Heat the olive oil in a large saucepan over medium-high heat. Add the tomatoes, roasted bell pepper, olives, lemon zest, vinegar, shallots, and parsley and sauté until the vegetables are tender. Add this mixture to the bowl of chickpeas, season with salt and pepper to taste, and set aside in a warm place.

Olive Oil–Poached Halibut with Black Chickpea Tapenade (continued)

Variation:

Karen Giblin and Dr. Mache Seibel suggest an alternative method of poaching the halibut used in this recipe:

1 quart water
½ medium-size onion, sliced
6 whole black peppercorns
3 tablespoons lemon juice
1 bay leaf
1 teaspoon salt
½ cup dry white wine or water

Combine all ingredients in large skillet or Dutch oven. Add enough liquid to cover the halibut during poaching. Simmer for 20–30 minutes to blend flavors.

Then, add the halibut; cover and simmer over low heat for 10–15 minutes, or until it flakes easily when tested with a fork. (Note: Avoid using high heat. Boiling action will break up fish.) Lift cooked halibut carefully from liquid with wide spatula. Drain well, patting excess moisture from fish with paper towels.

To make the fish, fill a saucepan (large enough to hold the fish in one layer) with the olive oil (enough to cover the fish), and heat to 130°F. Add the fish and poach for about 10 minutes, until the fish is cooked through. Place the fish in a serving dish and cover with the chickpea tapenade. Serve immediately.

—*Chef Neal Fraser*

Per serving (Chef Fraser's version): 6,040 Cal.; 45 GI; 67 g Prot.; 60 g Carb.; 87 g SFA; 451 g MUFA; 68 g PUFA; 6 g Omega-3; 170 mg Calc.; 2,863 mg Sod.; 1,810 mg Pot.; 11 mg Iron; 2 mg Phytoestrogen; 15 g Fiber

Sweet-and-Sour Tuna

Tuna is the number-one fish in Sicily. This recipe, called tonno agrodolce, *is common to the island's cuisine. Sweet and sour in taste and served rare, it's sure to become your favorite way of making tuna. Tuna is full of omega-3 fatty acids, which help lower our risk of cardiovascular disease. It's also beneficial to our skin and is a good source of selenium, important to our liver's health.*

Yield: 4 servings

4 tuna steaks
All-purpose flour, for coating
Salt
3 tablespoons extra-virgin olive oil
1 large onion, sliced
½ cup red wine vinegar
3 tablespoons Marsala
½ cup golden raisins
12 large pitted green olives
3 bay leaves

Rinse the tuna steaks, pat dry, and then coat them with the flour and salt.

Heat the olive oil in a large skillet over medium heat. Add the onion and sauté until tender but not browned. Add the tuna steaks and cook for 4 minutes on each side. Add the vinegar, Marsala, raisins, olives, and bay leaves and cook for an additional 7 minutes. Turn off the heat, cover the skillet, and let rest for 10 minutes, for the flavor of the sauce to be absorbed by the tuna. Before serving, discard the bay leaves.

—*Karen's Cucina*

Per serving: 282 Cal.; 63 GI; 18 g Prot.; 20 g Carb.; 2 g SFA; 9 g MUFA; 2 g PUFA; 0.5 g Omega-3; 47 mg Calc.; 556 mg Sod.; 459 mg Pot.; 1 mg Iron; 0.34 mg Phytoestrogen; 2 g Fiber

Swordfish with Orange-Lemon Sauce

This recipe not only looks fantastic, it also tastes fantastic. There are genuine health benefits to eating swordfish because of the omega-3 fatty acids that may ward off heart disease and strokes. Fish also contains selenium, antioxidants, and protein.

Yield: 4 servings

4 swordfish steaks

½ cup freshly squeezed lemon juice

½ cup freshly squeezed orange juice

1 cup finely chopped onion

3 cloves garlic, chopped finely

Handful of chopped Italian (flat-leaf) parsley

Zest of 1 lemon

Zest of 1 orange

Salt and pepper

Preheat the oven to 375°F.

Place the swordfish steaks in a glass baking dish. Add the lemon and orange juices, onion, garlic, parsley, lemon and orange zest, and salt and pepper. Turn the swordfish steaks to ensure they are well coated and bake for 20 minutes.

Serve with the sauce spooned over the top of the fish.

—*Karen's Cucina*

Per serving: 268 Cal.; 51 GI; 34 g Prot.; 11 g Carb.; 2 g SFA; 3 g MUFA; 3 g PUFA; 2 g Omega-3; 46 mg Calc.; 98 mg Sod.; 965 mg Pot.; 1 mg Iron; 0.08 mg Phytoestrogen; 1 g Fiber

Halibut in Wine and Tomatoes

This halibut has a succulent sauce and is surprisingly simple and elegant. Fish and tomatoes are a combination that optimizes our health.

Yield: 4 servings

¼ cup olive oil

1 cup chopped onion

3 cloves garlic, sliced thinly

Pinch of red pepper flakes

4 (6-ounce) halibut fillets

1 (28-ounce) can tomatoes

1 cup dry white wine

⅓ cup chopped fresh Italian (flat-leaf) parsley

Salt and pepper

Heat the olive oil in a large saucepan over medium-high heat. Add the onion, garlic, and red pepper flakes and sauté until the onion is tender. Lower the heat to medium and add the halibut, tomatoes, and wine. Cover and cook for 8 minutes. Stir in the parsley and salt and pepper to taste and serve.

—*Karen's Cucina*

Per serving: 378 Cal.; 55 GI; 34 g Prot.; 14 g Carb.; 2 g SFA; 10 g MUFA; 2 g PUFA; 1 g Omega-3; 111 mg Calc.; 431 mg Sod.; 971 mg Pot.; 3 mg Iron; 0.032 mg Phytoestrogen; 3 g Fiber

Avoid Skipping Meals

Skipping meals can affect your memory and concentration. Remember when your mom said, "You can't start your day on an empty stomach"? She was right. Antioxidant-rich foods such as blueberries and vegetables help slow down those memory lapses.

Cod with Rosemary and Anchovies

This recipe is very quick and easy to make, has fantastic flavors, and is delicious and nutritious as well. It's also an excellent source of protein, omega-3 fatty acids, and vitamins B_6 and B_{12}. Rosemary contains antioxidants and vitamin E.

Yield: 4 servings

3 tablespoons olive oil

I (2-ounce) can anchovy fillets

I (3- to 4-pound) whole codfish

4 sprigs of fresh rosemary, plus extra, chopped

4 fresh basil leaves, torn, plus extra, chopped

½ cup bread crumbs

Salt and pepper

I cup pitted black olives

Preheat the oven to 400°F. With olive oil, lightly grease a baking dish large enough to hold the fish.

Heat 2 tablespoons of the olive oil in a small skillet over medium-low heat. Add the anchovies, mashing them with a wooden spoon, and cook them until they almost disintegrate. Set aside.

Place the codfish in the greased baking dish and spoon half the anchovies inside the cavity. Add the rosemary sprigs and torn basil leaves, and drizzle the remaining tablespoon of olive oil over the fish. Spoon the remaining anchovies over the fish and sprinkle with the chopped rosemary and basil and the bread crumbs. Season with salt and pepper and bake, uncovered, for 30 minutes. Serve with the olives.

—Karen's Cucina

Per serving: 530 Cal.; 70 GI; 70 g Prot.; 12 g Carb.; 3 g SFA; 12 g MUFA; 4 g PUFA; 2 g Omega-3; 142 mg Calc.; 1,251 mg Sod.; 1,023 mg Pot.; 4 mg Iron; 0.1 mg Phytoestrogen; 2 g Fiber

Red Snapper with Tomatoes

This is an incredibly simple recipe with a Mediterranean flair, fragrant and delicious with a great gourmet taste. Red snapper is high in protein yet low in fat.

Yield: 6 servings

3 tablespoons extra-virgin olive oil

2 cloves garlic, sliced thinly

1 (16-ounce) can Italian tomatoes

Salt and pepper

2½ pounds red snapper fillets

Handful of chopped fresh Italian (flat-leaf) parsley

Red Hot Ingredient: Red Snapper

- Vitamins B_6 and B_{12}
- Phosphorus, potassium, and selenium
- Protein
- Omega-3 fatty acids

Heat the olive oil in a large skillet over low heat. Add the garlic and cook for about 3 minutes, until the garlic is tender. Add the tomatoes (mashing them with a wooden spoon) and salt and pepper to taste and cook for an additional 10 minutes. Add the red snapper and simmer for 20 minutes longer on one side only (do not turn the fish over). Sprinkle with the parsley and serve.

—*Karen's Cucina*

Per serving: 375 Cal.; 50 GI; 55 g Prot.; 6 g Carb.; 2 g SFA; 8 g MUFA; 2 g PUFA; 1 g Omega-3; 98 mg Calc.; 403 mg Sod.; 1,063 mg Pot.; 3 mg Iron; 0 mg Phytoestrogen; 2 g Fiber

Salmon with Pomegranate Caponata and Fennel Slaw

Salmon is one of the richest sources of omega-3s, the king of fish oils. Eating salmon helps to keep our arteries clear and our heart strong. Pomegranate seeds are full of anti-oxidants and fiber. This recipe is not only tasty and unique, but it's healthy as well.

Yield: 4 servings

Caponata:

2 tablespoons olive oil

2 cloves garlic, minced

2 tablespoons minced shallots

2 tablespoons peeled and minced fresh ginger

½ cup pomegranate seeds

2 tablespoons nonpareil capers, strained

1 tablespoon freshly squeezed lemon juice

2 tablespoons finely chopped fresh cilantro

2 tablespoons finely chopped fresh Italian (flat-leaf) parsley

Salt and pepper

Fennel Slaw:

1 head fennel, cored and sliced paper thin

2 tablespoons olive oil

Juice of 1 lemon

2 tablespoons snipped fresh dill

Salt and pepper

Salmon:

2 tablespoons grapeseed oil

4 (6-ounce) wild salmon fillets (preferably with the skin)

Salt and pepper

Per serving: 409 Cal.; 51 GI; 38 g Prot.; 6 g Carb.; 3 g SFA; 10 g MUFA; 8 g PUFA; 2 g Omega-3; 24 mg Calc.; 234 mg Sod.; 718 mg Pot.; 1 mg Iron; 0 mg Phytoestrogen; 1 g Fiber

To make the caponata, heat the oil in a small skillet over medium heat. Add the garlic, shallots, and ginger and sauté for 4 minutes, until tender. Stir in the pomegranate seeds and remove from the heat. Mix in the capers, lemon juice, cilantro, and parsley and season with salt and pepper to taste. Set aside.

To make the fennel slaw, combine the fennel, olive oil, lemon juice, dill, and salt and pepper to taste in a large bowl. Mix well and set aside.

To make the salmon, preheat the oven to 375°F. Lightly grease a baking dish.

Heat the grapeseed oil in a skillet over medium-high heat.

Season the salmon fillets with salt and pepper and place them in the skillet, skin side down, and cook until golden. Then place the fillets in the greased baking dish, keeping the skin side down, and bake for 5 minutes for medium rare to medium.

To serve, spoon the fennel slaw onto four individual serving plates, place a fillet of fish on top of each salad, and top with the caponata.

—Michelle Bernstein

Wild Alaskan Halibut Crusted with Brioche with a Salad of French Green Beans, Belgian Endive, Watercress, and Tomatoes

This is a delicious early spring and summer dish to enjoy! The colorful array of vegetables in this dish offers a wide range of vitamins, minerals, fiber, and phytochemicals that may reduce our risk of cancer and heart disease.

Yield: 2 servings

Salad:

½ pound French green beans, trimmed

2 Roma tomatoes

2 white Belgian endives

1 bunch of watercress (tender leaf or hydroponic)

Salt and freshly ground pepper

2 tablespoons hazelnut oil

2 teaspoons sherry wine vinegar

Halibut:

½ pound brioche bread

¼ cup unsalted butter (½ stick)

2 (7-ounce) wild Alaskan halibut fillets

Salt and cracked pepper

To make the salad, in a pot of boiling salted water, blanch the beans, remove from the water with a slotted spoon, and refresh them in ice-cold water. Set aside and keep the water boiling. Core the tomatoes and score a small X on the top of each tomato. Place them in the boiling water and blanch them for a moment, lift them out with a slotted spoon and refresh under cold running water, and then, with a sharp knife, peel away and discard the skin. Cut off the top of the tomatoes in a petal shape (reserve tops to use as a garnish) and scoop out and discard the seeds. Cut the tomatoes into julienne strips and set aside.

Split the endives in half, core them, and then cut them into julienne strips. Place a wet paper towel on top and set aside.

Place the endives, tomatoes, beans, and watercress in a salad bowl. Season to taste with the salt and freshly ground pepper and set the salad aside. Whisk together the oil and vinegar and set aside.

Wild Alaskan Halibut Crusted with Brioche with a Salad . . . (continued)

To make the fish, cut up the brioche and toast until lightly golden brown, and then place in a food processor and process to make bread crumbs. Set aside on a plate.

Clarify the butter by melting it in a small saucepan over low heat. Skim off the foam that rises to the top, and once the solids settle in the bottom, remove the clear butter and discard the milk solids. Keep the clarified butter warm.

Season the halibut fillets with salt and cracked pepper and set aside. Put half the clarified butter in a nonstick or stainless-steel skillet and heat over medium-high heat. Dip the fish fillets into the remaining clarified butter, and then into the brioche crumbs.

Lower the heat to medium and place the fillets in the skillet. Cook for about 3 minutes on each side, until golden brown on both sides. (If the fillets are very thick, place them in a 375°F oven and bake for 5 minutes to cook through.) Remove the fish from the skillet and let them rest on a paper towel to remove the excess fat.

To serve, toss the oil and vinegar dressing with the salad, place the fish on individual serving plates, top each with the salad, garnish each with a tomato top, and serve!

—*Carrie Nahabedian*

Per serving: 965 Cal.; 66 GI; 56 g Prot.; 66 g Carb.; 22 g SFA; 23 g MUFA; 6 g PUFA; 1 g Omega-3; 132 mg Calc.; 437 mg Sod.; 1,061 mg Pot.; 5 mg Iron; 1 mg Phytoestrogen; 6 g Fiber

If you can't find Alaskan halibut, you can use any white-fleshed fish. You can use brioche buns, rolls, or a loaf. Extra-virgin olive oil can be substituted for the hazelnut oil. Sherry wine vinegar has a mild and distinctive flavor; however you may use red wine vinegar instead. Pole beans may be substituted for the French green beans.

Wild Snapper Mediterranean with Artichokes à la Barigoule, Valencia Oranges, French Green Beans, and Basil

The fresh vegetables and mild seasonings in this recipe complement the depth of flavor of the snapper without overpowering the sweetness. The presentation of the dish is just as impressive as the taste! Artichokes may help reduce cholesterol, relieve irritable bowel syndrome symptoms, and stabilize blood sugar levels in diabetes.

Yield: 4 servings

2 artichokes

2 tablespoons salt

½ lemon

7 tablespoons olive oil

1 leek, white with a touch of green, split, cleaned, and cut into ¼-inch slices

½ medium-size yellow onion, halved and sliced thinly

1 rib celery, sliced thinly

1 carrot, peeled, channel cut, and sliced thinly

Salt and cracked peppercorns, plus 5 whole peppercorns

¼ cup white wine

1 bay leaf

A few sprigs of fresh thyme

A few sprigs of fresh parsley

4 cloves garlic

4 (4- to 5-ounce) red snapper fillets, skin on

½ pound French green beans, blanched

2 tomatoes, peeled, seeded, and sliced thinly

2 Valencia oranges, peeled and segmented

3 sprigs of fresh basil, cut into long, thin strips

All the vegetables are for garnish and should be cut with care and attention.

Trim and clean the artichokes, leaving the bottom and heart intact. Place the artichokes in a deep stainless-steel saucepan with fresh cold water to cover and the salt and half lemon.

Cover with a white napkin or cloth and cook over medium-high heat until tender. Remove the artichokes from the water and cool immediately under cold running water. Cut the artichokes in half, remove and discard the chokes, and then cut the artichokes into quarters. Set aside.

Heat 3 tablespoons of the olive oil in a large, heavy saucepan over low heat. Add the leek, onion, celery, and carrot and cover the saucepan and sweat the vegetables until they are just tender. Season with salt and cracked peppercorns to taste, and then add 1¼ cups of water and the white wine to cover the vegetables.

Make a bouquet garni by tying the bay leaf, thyme sprigs, whole peppercorns, and parsley stems in a cheesecloth bag and place it in the saucepan. Bring to a boil, and then

Wild Snapper Mediterranean . . . (continued)

lower the heat and simmer the *barigoule* over medium heat until the carrots are tender. Remove from the heat and place the pan in an ice bath to cool.

Place the garlic cloves in a small saucepan, cover with water, and bring to a quick boil. Refresh under cold water and repeat the process three times. In the final cooking, add ½ teaspoon of salt. Cool the now "sweet" garlic cloves under cold water, slice thinly, and set aside.

Heat 1 tablespoon of the olive oil in a nonstick or heavy skillet over medium-high heat. Season the fish fillets with salt and pepper and place, flesh side down, in the skillet. Sear the fish for about 2 minutes, or until golden brown, and then turn and cook on the skin side for an additional 3 minutes. With a spoon, baste the fish with the olive oil and cooking juices for added flavor and color. Set aside and keep warm.

To finish the beautiful dish, pour the barigoule broth and vegetables into a casserole. Bring to a boil, lower the heat, and stir in the remaining 3 tablespoons of olive oil. Garnish with the artichokes, French green beans, tomatoes, sweet garlic, Valencia oranges, and basil. Place the fish in a deep bowl, spoon the barigoule over the top, and serve immediately.

—*Carrie Nahabedian*

Per serving: 342 Cal.; 48 GI; 11 g Prot.; 29 g Carb.; 3 g SFA; 15 g MUFA; 2 g PUFA; 0.4 g Omega-3; 107 mg Calc.; 89 mg Sod.; 782 mg Pot.; 2 mg Iron; 0 mg Phytoestrogen; 10 g Fiber

Red Hot Ingredient: Artichokes

- Vitamins A and C, niacin, and folic acid
- Chromium, magnesium, manganese, and potassium
- Antioxidants
- Fiber

Soy-Grilled Salmon Skewers

This delicious salmon recipe is easy to prepare and impressive looking for dinner guests. You can buy furikake *(seaweed and sesame rice seasoning) in the Asian section at most grocery stores. It is available vegetarian style or with dehydrated egg or shrimp. Salmon is one of the healthiest fish to eat: It contains lots of minerals that may be beneficial for our cardiovascular and eye health, and even our skin and hair. Substitute low-sodium soy sauce to lower the sodium content of this recipe.*

Yield: 4 servings

1 (1-pound) salmon fillet, sliced lengthwise into 4 (1-inch) strips
½ cup soy sauce
½ cup freshly squeezed orange juice
¼ cup freshly squeezed lime juice
1 tablespoon minced ginger
1 clove garlic, minced
1 teaspoon red pepper flakes
1 teaspoon *furikake*

Red Hot Ingredient: Salmon

- Vitamins A, B, and D
- Protein
- Omega-3 fatty acids

Soak four bamboo skewers in water for 30 minutes, then thread each salmon strip onto a soaked skewer and place in a shallow dish.

In a bowl, whisk together the soy sauce, orange juice, lime juice, ginger, garlic, red pepper flakes, and *furikake*. Pour ½ cup of the soy mixture over the skewers, turning to coat. Let marinate for 30 minutes. Reserve the remaining marinade for dipping.

Preheat an outdoor grill to medium-high heat. Oil your grill generously, and then cook the skewers for 2 minutes per side, brushing often with the marinade, or until the fish starts to flake. Let them rest for 2 minutes before serving. Serve with the reserved marinade on the side.

—Donnie Ferneau Jr., CEC

Per serving: 200 Cal.; 45 GI; 27 g Prot.; 8 g Carb.; 2 g SFA; 2 g MUFA; 2 g PUFA; 1.5 g Omega-3; 26 mg Calc.; 1,866 mg Sod.; 732 mg Pot.; 1.5 mg Iron; 0.6 mg Phytoestrogen; 1 g Fiber

Broiled George's Bank Codfish with Citrus and Fennel Slaw

This is a favorite dish at the Black Dog Café on Martha's Vineyard that you can make at home. It's delicious and light and doesn't take long to prepare. For convenience, you can make the slaw the day before and refrigerate until the fish is cooked. Fennel, citrus fruit, plus omega-3 cod is surely a recipe for good health.

Yield: 4 servings

Slaw:
1 cup fennel, shaved paper thin
1 tablespoon chopped fennel fronds (tops)
3 navel oranges, segmented
1 pink grapefruit, segmented
1 tablespoon fennel seeds, toasted
2 tablespoons olive oil
2 tablespoons sherry vinegar
1 teaspoon whole-grain mustard

Fish:
4 (8-ounce) cod fillets
Salt and pepper
¼ cup dry white wine
2 tablespoons lemon juice

To make the slaw, place the fennel shavings and fronds, orange and grapefruit segments, and fennel seeds in a salad bowl. In a small bowl, whisk together the olive oil, vinegar, and mustard and toss with the fennel mixture. Set aside.

To make the fish, preheat the oven to 350°F. Place the codfish in a shallow baking dish and season with salt and pepper. Pour the wine and lemon juice over the top and bake for 8 to 10 minutes, until opaque. Serve immediately with the slaw.

—*Chef Bill Hart*

Per serving (fish): 148 Cal.; 36 GI; 2 g Prot.; 21 g Carb.; 1 g SFA; 5 g MUFA; 1 g PUFA; 0 g Omega-3; 83 mg Calc.; 46 mg Sod.; 390 mg Pot.; 0.6 mg Iron; 0 mg Phytoestrogen; 5 g Fiber

Per serving (slaw): 221 Cal.; 45 GI; 42 g Prot.; 1 g Carb.; 0.6 g SFA; 0.4 g MUFA; 1 g PUFA; 1 g Omega-3; 34 mg Calc.; 187 mg Sod.; 628 mg Pot.; 0.6 mg Iron; 0 mg Phytoestrogen; 0 g Fiber

Hamachi en Escabeche

This recipe has gotten rave reviews from many restaurant critics. Tuna supplies a variety of important nutrients for our health.

Yield: 4 servings

Ajo Blanco Puree:
¼ cup extra-virgin olive oil
6 cloves garlic, sliced thinly
2 fresh basil leaves
¼ cup sliced baguette, crusts removed
½ cup roasted Marcona almonds
2 cups spring water
1 tablespoon kosher salt
1 tablespoon aged sherry
1 teaspoon vinegar

Black Olive Escabeche:
¼ cup pitted kalamata olives
¼ cup honey
¼ cup white wine vinegar
3 sprigs of fresh thyme, leaves chopped
2 shallots, chopped very finely
¼ cup extra-virgin olive oil
1½ teaspoons kosher salt
¼ teaspoon freshly ground pepper
¼ bunch of parsley, chopped
5 cloves garlic, roasted and mashed

Hamachi:
12 cucumber blossoms
½ cup black olive escabeche (above)
¼ cup blended oil
1 (12-ounce) hamachi loin (yellowtail tuna)
Kosher salt and freshly ground pepper
½ cup ajo blanco puree (above)

To make the ajo blanco puree, heat the olive oil in a small saucepan over medium-low heat. Add the garlic and basil and sauté until the garlic turns light golden. Remove from the heat and discard the basil. Add the sliced baguette to the oil and let soak for a few minutes. When the oil mixture is cool, place it in a food processor with the almonds, spring water, salt, sherry, and vinegar and puree for at least 5 minutes. Strain through a fine-mesh strainer and chill for at least 4 hours, or until the puree is thick and mousselike.

To make the black olive escabeche, combine all the ingredients, mix well, and refrigerate.

To assemble the dish, toss the cucumber blossoms with ½ cup of the black olive escabeche and let it marinate for at least 5 minutes. Heat the blended oil in a skillet over high heat.

Season the hamachi loin generously with salt and pepper and place in the skillet. Sear the hamachi on one side until lightly caramelized but still raw. Remove from the heat and slice the fish into four equal pieces. Place 2 tablespoons of the ajo blanco puree on each of four individual serving plates. Place a slice of fish on top of the puree. Spoon three cucumber blossoms and one-quarter of the remaining black olive escabeche mixture on and around each serving of fish. Serve immediately.

—*Chef de Cuisine Michael Fiorello*

Per serving: 581 Cal.; 61 GI; 25 g Prot.; 30 g Carb.; 5 g SFA; 26 g MUFA; 6 g PUFA; 1 g Omega-3; 127 mg Calc.; 1,009 mg Sod.; 523 mg Pot.; 4 mg Iron; 0 mg Phytoestrogen; 4 g Fiber

Sautéed Day-Boat Scallops, Nettles, Sunchokes, and Raisin-Caper Emulsion

Impress your guests with this sophisticated entrée that includes the finest of ingredients. The nettle plant is often considered a wonder plant because of its health benefits. In the past, nettles have been used as remedies for allergies, anemia, and kidney diseases. Cook nettles as you would spinach (they taste and look similar).

Yield: 4 servings

Nettles:

4 ounces nettles, stems removed (wear gloves)

2 tablespoons olive oil

¼ cup water

Kosher salt

Sunchokes:

2 tablespoons olive oil

2 sunchokes (Jerusalem artichokes), peeled and sliced with a mandoline slicer

Kosher salt

Raisin-Caper Sauce:

⅔ cup sultana (golden) raisins

2 tablespoons capers

2 tablespoons sherry wine vinegar

½ cup water

Scallops:

4 large (size U-10) dry-packed day-boat scallops

Kosher salt

1 tablespoon canola oil

2 tablespoons butter

To prepare the nettles (make sure you wear gloves when handling nettles, as they will sting your hands), in a saucepan, combine the nettles, olive oil, water, and salt and cook over medium-low heat for about 10 minutes, until the nettles are tender. Set aside.

To prepare the sunchokes, heat the olive oil in a skillet over medium-high heat. Add the sunchokes and sauté until golden brown. Season with salt to taste and set aside.

To make the sauce, put the raisins, capers, vinegar, and water in a saucepan and simmer until the raisins are rehydrated. If the mixture becomes too dry, add some more water. Blend in a food processor and set aside.

Sautéed Day-Boat Scallops, Nettles, Sunchokes, and Raisin-Caper Emulsion (continued)

> ## Red Hot Ingredient: Nettles
>
> - Vitamins A, C, and E
> - Boron, calcium, and iron
> - Beta-carotene
> - Phosphates

To make the scallops, season them with salt. Heat a skillet over high heat until hot, add the canola oil, and immediately add the scallops. Sauté for 30 seconds. Add the butter and continue to cook until the bottom side of the scallops are golden brown. Flip the scallops, lower the heat, and cook for another 2 minutes. Remove from the skillet and pat dry.

To serve, spoon the sauce onto each of four individual serving plates, then the nettles, then the scallops, and top each with the sunchokes. Serve immediately.

—Chef Neal Fraser

Per serving: 318 Cal.; 61 GI; 6 g Prot.; 29 g Carb.; 2 g SFA; 15 g MUFA; 3 g PUFA; 0.8 g Omega-3; 97 mg Calc.; 853 mg Sod.; 512 mg Pot.; 2 mg Iron; 0.052 mg Phytoestrogen; 3 g Fiber

Orange Scallops

This is an incredibly simple recipe with a Mediterranean flair, and it's fragrant and delicious with a great gourmet taste. Scallops are low in fat yet have a high amount of protein.

Yield: 4 servings

4 tablespoons extra-virgin olive oil

3 cloves garlic, chopped finely

1 leek, trimmed, rinsed, and sliced thinly

1 (28-ounce) can tomatoes, chopped

Pinch of salt

1 teaspoon orange zest

Pinch of cayenne

1 pound sea scallops

½ cup all-purpose flour

Heat 3 tablespoons of the olive oil in a medium-size saucepan over medium heat. Add the garlic and leek and sauté for about 10 minutes, until the leek is tender. Add the tomatoes with their juice, the salt, orange zest, and cayenne and bring to a boil. Lower the heat and simmer for about 7 minutes, until the sauce begins to thicken.

Rinse the scallops and pat dry, and then coat them lightly with the flour. If the scallops are large, cut them in half.

In a large skillet, heat the remaining 1 tablespoon of olive oil over medium-high heat. Add the scallops and sauté until lightly golden. Stir in the sauce mixture and cook for about 3 minutes, until heated through. Add salt if needed.

—*Karen's Cucina*

Per serving: 248 Cal.; 63 GI; 16 g Prot.; 21 g Carb.; 2 g SFA; 7 g MUFA; 1.5 g PUFA; 0.3 g Omega-3; 135 mg Calc.; 730 mg Sod.; 674 mg Pot.; 4 mg Iron; 0 mg Phytoestrogen; 3 g Fiber

Shrimp in Tomato Sauce with Capers

This is a delicious and aromatic Sicilian dish with a combination of excellent ingredients to benefit your health. Your guests will want this recipe, for sure.

Yield: 4 servings

1½ pounds shrimp

½ cup extra-virgin olive oil

1 medium-size red onion, chopped finely

3 cloves garlic, chopped finely

1 large rib celery, chopped finely

1 small carrot, pared and chopped finely

1 (28-ounce) can Italian tomatoes

Salt and pepper

5 tablespoons raisins

5 tablespoons pine nuts

6 tablespoons capers, drained

6 bay leaves

Handful of chopped fresh basil

Handful of chopped fresh Italian (flat-leaf) parsley

1 lemon, cut into 4 wedges

Red Hot Ingredient: Shrimp

- Vitamins B_{12} and D
- Selenium
- Protein
- Omega-3 fatty acids

Per serving: 533 Cal.; 55 GI; 31 g Prot.; 26 g Carb.; 5 g SFA; 22 g MUFA; 7 g PUFA; 1 g Omega-3; 168 mg Calc.; 1,205 mg Sod.; 960 mg Pot.; 8 mg Iron; 0.028 mg Phytoestrogen; 5 g Fiber

Preheat the oven to 375°F.

Wash and drain the shrimp. Set aside in ice-cold water.

Heat the olive oil in a medium-size skillet over medium heat. Add the onion, garlic, celery, and carrot and sauté for 10 minutes, until the vegetables are tender. Add the tomatoes, smashing them with a wooden spoon, and cook for 15 minutes longer. Season with salt and pepper to taste.

Meanwhile, soak the raisins in small bowl of warm water for 10 minutes, then drain them. Add them and the pine nuts and capers to the skillet and cook for an additional 10 minutes.

Transfer the tomato mixture to a glass baking dish. Drain the shrimp and place them over the tomato sauce, and then place the bay leaves over the shrimp. Cover the baking dish with aluminum foil and bake for 10 minutes. Remove the dish from the oven, discard the bay leaves, and gently mix the shrimp into the tomato sauce.

Serve sprinkled with the basil and parsley and with the lemon wedges on the side.

—Karen's Cucina

Seafood Couscous Paella

Whole wheat couscous soaks up the savory saffron-infused broth in this paella, a classic dish exemplifying the Mediterranean diet. Loaded with an abundance of fish, which the American Heart Association recommends eating at least twice per week, this recipe will boost your intake of omega-3 fatty acids, which can lower cholesterol. Save some for leftovers and you'll be set for the week!

Yield: 4 servings

4 tablespoons extra-virgin olive oil

2 medium-size onions, chopped

2 cloves garlic, minced

2 teaspoons dried thyme

I teaspoon ground fennel

I teaspoon kosher salt

Pinch of white pepper

2 pinches of saffron

2 cups diced canned tomatoes and their juice

½ cup vegetable broth

½ pound bay scallops

½ pound small bay shrimp, peeled and deveined

I cup whole wheat couscous

Heat the olive oil in a large saucepan over medium heat.

Add the onions and garlic and sauté for 3 to 4 minutes, until tender but not browned. Add the thyme, fennel, salt, pepper, and saffron and cook for a few minutes longer. Stir in the tomatoes and broth and bring to a boil. Lower the heat and simmer, covered, for 5 minutes. Increase the heat again to medium and stir in the scallops and shrimp. Cook for 6 to 8 minutes, stirring occasionally. Stir in the couscous, cover, and remove from heat. Let stand for 5 minutes, until the couscous is tender. Fluff with a large fork and serve immediately.

—Chef Aldo

Per serving: 399 Cal.; 61 GI; 22 g Prot.; 43 g Carb.; 2 g SFA; 10 g MUFA; 2 g PUFA; 0.3 g Omega-3; 88 mg Calc.; 806 mg Sod.; 589 mg Pot.; 3 mg Iron; 0 mg Phytoestrogen; 4 g Fiber

Variation:

Halibut, Dover sole, and red snapper also work well in this dish, instead of the scallops and shrimp.

Seared Hand-Harvested Maine Sea Scallops with Caramelized Onions, Savoy Cabbage, French Lentils, and Balsamic Syrup

You can obtain fresh diver sea scallops from a high-quality fish source. If these are unavailable, use the fresh sea scallops (try to get the U-10 size) at your local grocery store. French du Puy lentils are green and a little smaller than the average lentil. They take a little longer to cook, but hold their shape well. Low in fat, high in protein and fiber, you can't go wrong with a good serving of lentils, as in this dish.

Yield: 8 scallops (2 servings)

2 pounds French du Puy or green lentils

Chicken broth or water

1 small carrot

1 rib celery

¼ onion

1 head savoy cabbage

½ cup olive oil

2 yellow onions, sliced thinly

Salt

2 cups balsamic vinegar

2 scallops per person as an appetizer or 4 as an entrée

Cracked peppercorns

½ bunch of fresh parsley, chopped

Put the lentils in a large saucepan and add chicken broth or water to cover. Stir in the carrot, celery, and onion and bring to a boil. Lower the heat and simmer, covered, for about 45 minutes, or until the lentils are tender.

Remove and discard the outer leaves of the cabbage, leaving the inner yellow leaves. Remove and discard the core and blanch the leaves in boiling salted water, and then refresh them in ice water. Cut the leaves into long, thin strips and set aside.

Heat the olive oil in a small skillet over high heat. Add the onions and sauté with care, stirring constantly, until the onions are glazed and caramelized. Season with salt to taste and set aside.

Continues . . .

Seared Hand-Harvested Maine Sea Scallops with Caramelized Onions . . . (continued)

In a heavy saucepan, reduce the balsamic vinegar over medium-high heat until it is the consistency of syrup. Take care not to burn the vinegar. Keep at room temperature or warmer if you are going to use it immediately. It can be refrigerated indefinitely and warmed up as needed.

Pat the scallops dry and season with salt and cracked pepper. Sear in a heavy skillet over medium-high to high heat, browning the scallops on all sides. (If necessary, they can be placed in a 350°F oven for a few minutes to complete cooking.)

Mix the onions and cabbage together, place on individual serving plates, and top each with some of the lentils. Place the scallops on top, and if there are any pan juices from the scallops, spoon a touch or two over each serving. Drizzle each dish with the balsamic syrup and garnish with the chopped parsley. Serve immediately.

—*Carrie Nahabedian*

Per serving: 1,190 Cal.; 27 GI; 72 g Prot.; 156 g Carb.; 4 g SFA; 21 g MUFA; 4 g PUFA; 0.7 g Omega-3; 255 mg Calc.; 219 mg Sod.; 2,937 mg Pot.; 24 mg Iron; 0.05 mg Phytoestrogen; 39 g Fiber

Lobster and Duck Chow Mein

Fortified with an abundance of fresh ingredients, this is a delectable new way to enjoy chow mein. Healthy, authentic Chinese food is much different than the takeout you commonly see at the mall. Meat is used here in moderation, prepared with polyunsaturated oils, and this dish does not use any milk-based ingredients. In traditional Chinese cooking, emphasis is given to rice, noodles, and vegetables. The lemongrass in this dish offers not only a distinct flavor but is also good for gas relief and digestion.

Yield: 4 servings

BBQ Duck Marinade:
2 cinnamon sticks
¼ cup coriander seeds
¼ cup star anise
5 cloves
5 whole allspice berries
½ teaspoon red pepper flakes
¼ cup Szechuan peppercorns
4 cups hoisin sauce
4 cups soy sauce
1½ cups sesame oil
1 cup rice wine vinegar
Zest of 2 oranges
1 stalk lemongrass
1 small bunch of green onions, chopped
1 tablespoon minced fresh ginger
1 tablespoon minced garlic
½ pound duck, cut into 4 pieces

Chow Mein Sauce:
1 cup Chinese barbecue sauce
1 cup oyster sauce
1½ cups hoisin sauce
½ cup black soy sauce
2 tablespoons *sambal oelek* (Indonesian seasoning paste)
¼ cup Thai sweet chili sauce
¼ cup sugar

Entrée:
1 tablespoon peanut oil
½ pound lobster (claw and knuckle), chopped
¾ cup julienned celery
¾ cup julienned carrots
½ pound shiitake mushrooms, sliced
4 teaspoons minced garlic
4 teaspoons minced shallots
4 teaspoons minced fresh ginger
24 ounces egg noodles, prepared per package instructions

Garnishes:
Bean sprouts
Garlic chives, chopped
Red bell pepper, seeded and julienned
Fresh cilantro, minced
Fresno pepper rings

Continues . . .

Lobster and Duck Chow Mein (continued)

To make the BBQ duck marinade, preheat the oven to 350°F.

Place the cinnamon, coriander, anise, cloves, allspice, red pepper flakes, and peppercorns on a baking sheet and toast in the oven for 2 minutes. Combine the hoisin sauce, soy sauce, sesame oil, and vinegar in a large bowl and mix well. Stir in the toasted spices, orange zest, lemongrass, green onions, ginger, and garlic. Add the duck pieces and marinate in the refrigerator for 12 to 24 hours.

To make the chow mein sauce, combine the barbecue sauce, oyster sauce, hoisin sauce, soy sauce, *sambal oelek,* chili sauce, ¼ cup of water, and the sugar in a large bowl. Mix well and set aside.

To make the entrée, remove the duck from the marinade and pat dry. Heat the peanut oil in a wok over high heat. Add the marinated duck and the lobster and sauté for 1 minute, and then move them to the side of the wok. Add the celery, carrots, mushrooms, garlic, shallot, and ginger and sauté until the vegetables are tender. Add the chow mein sauce and the cooked noodles and sauté for 1 minute longer, stirring constantly. Garnish with the bean sprouts, chives, bell pepper, cilantro, and pepper rings. Serve immediately.

—Chef Brad Parsons

Per serving (about 2 tablespoons) (BBQ duck marinade): 254 Cal.; 84 GI; 4.5 g Prot.; 24 g Carb.; 2 g SFA; 6 g MUFA; 6 g PUFA; 1 g Omega-3; 42 mg Calc.; 3,087 mg Sod.; 197 mg Pot.; 2 mg Iron; 5 mg Phytoestrogen; 2 g Fiber

Per serving (about 2 tablespoons) (chow mein sauce): 68 Cal.; 79 GI; 1 g Prot.; 14 g Carb.; 0.1 g SFA; 0.1 g MUFA; 0.2 g PUFA; 0 g Omega-3; 17 mg Calc.; 1,055 mg Sod.; 112 mg Pot.; 0.5 mg Iron; 1.5 mg Phytoestrogen; 1 g Fiber

Per serving (entrée): 600 Cal.; 41 GI; 37 g Prot.; 89 g Carb.; 2 g SFA; 3 g MUFA; 3 g PUFA; 0.2 g Omega-3; 104 mg Calc.; 281 mg Sod.; 676 mg Pot.; 6 mg Iron; 0 mg Phytoestrogen; 6 g Fiber

What Happens to Your Body When You Eat a Large Meal?

The body's digestion brings blood into the abdomen, raises body temperature, and voilà, tells the hypothalamus part of the brain to send a signal that causes hot flashes. Eating smaller meals can help reduce the number of hot flashes.

Chicken and Shrimp Sorentina

Treat yourself to one of Liberatore's delicious and time-tested recipes. Use organic, skinless chicken breasts, which provide lean protein, niacin, lots of B vitamins, selenium, and other nutrients, without the additives, preservatives, or antibiotics.

Yield: 4 servings

4 boneless chicken breasts, pounded thin

All-purpose flour, for dredging

1 tablespoon margarine

10 to 12 jumbo shrimp

16 to 20 artichoke hearts, quartered

1 ripe tomato, diced

1½ teaspoons rubbed sage

1 tablespoon dried parsley

1 cup dry white wine

1 cup chicken broth

Salt and pepper

8 slices prosciutto

8 slices mozzarella cheese

Dredge the chicken in the flour. Heat the margarine in a large skillet over medium heat. Add the chicken and shrimp and sauté until the chicken is browned on one side. Add the artichoke hearts and tomatoes. Turn the chicken breasts and brown on the other side. Add the sage, parsley, and wine and simmer for 4 to 5 minutes. Add the broth, lower the heat to low, and simmer for a few minutes more. Season with salt and pepper to taste. Top with the prosciutto and mozzarella and continue to simmer until the cheese melts. Serve with lots of love over linguine and enjoy!

—*John Liberatore*

Per serving: 509 Cal.; 49 GI; 57 g Prot.; 26 g Carb.; 6 g SFA; 5 g MUFA; 2 g PUFA; 0.4 g Omega-3; 289 mg Calc.; 1,570 mg Sod.; 1,186 mg Pot.; 4 mg Iron; 0 mg Phytoestrogen; 16 g Fiber

Chicken Giovanni

This is a delicious low-calorie, low-fat dish that you will enjoy making and eating, and you'll plan on making it again. One cup of spinach only has about 40 calories, so you can't overdo it.

Yield: 2 servings

1 tablespoon margarine

2 boneless, skinless chicken breasts

All-purpose flour, for dusting chicken

2 sprigs of fresh rosemary

¼ cup white wine

¼ cup sherry wine

Juice of ½ lemon

½ cup chicken broth

¾ cup chopped spinach, well washed

Salt and pepper

2 slices mozzarella cheese

Melt the margarine in a skillet over medium-high heat. Lightly dust the chicken breasts with the flour and place in the skillet. Add the rosemary sprigs. Lightly brown the chicken on both sides. Add the wines and lemon juice. Lower the heat and simmer for 8 to 9 minutes. Add the broth and let simmer for an additional 8 to 9 minutes to reduce the broth.

Meanwhile, steam or boil the spinach until tender, and when the chicken is almost done, season with salt and pepper to taste and place half the spinach on top of each chicken breast. Top each with a slice of mozzarella and melt. Serve immediately.

—*John Liberatore*

Per serving: 360 Cal.; 59 GI; 34 g Prot.; 15 g Carb.; 4 g SFA; 4 g MUFA; 3 g PUFA; 0.4 g Omega-3; 189 mg Calc.; 333 mg Sod.; 678 mg Pot.; 3 mg Iron; 0 mg Phytoestrogen; 2 g Fiber

Curried Chicken

The aroma of this easy-to-prepare recipe will make your guests think you spent hours in the kitchen. Think about all the nutrients found in the wonderful spices used in this dish! Turmeric, the main ingredient in curry, is commonly used as an antiseptic in India and has long been associated with healing properties.

Yield: 4 servings

2 cups raw rice

1 tablespoon curry powder

1 tablespoon ground cinnamon

1 teaspoon ground ginger

¼ teaspoon red pepper flakes

2 tablespoons olive oil

1 onion, chopped

3 to 4 boneless chicken breasts, cut into bite-size pieces

2 to 3 heads broccoli

1 cube low-sodium chicken bouillon

1 (8-ounce) can reduced-fat coconut milk

1 tablespoon minced garlic

Salt and pepper

Cook the rice according to the package instructions and set aside.

In a small bowl, combine the curry, cinnamon, ginger, and red pepper flakes and set aside.

Heat the oil in a large saucepan over medium-high heat. Add the onion and chicken and cook until the chicken is done.

Meanwhile, steam the broccoli until tender.

When the chicken is done, add the spices, bouillon cube, and coconut milk to the chicken. Bring to a gentle boil, add the broccoli, and cook to heat through. Add salt and pepper to taste. Serve over the cooked rice.

—Cynthia Niles

Per serving: 557 Cal.; 54 GI; 36 g Prot.; 84 g Carb.; 2 g SFA; 3 g MUFA; 3 g PUFA; 0.2 g Omega-3; 208 mg Calc.; 151 mg Sod.; 609 mg Pot.; 4 mg Iron; 11 mg Phytoestrogen; 14 g Fiber

Moroccan Chicken over Apricot-Cranberry Couscous

The exciting spices in this recipe will fill your kitchen with a wonderfully savory aroma. Apricot-cranberry couscous is a sweet, healthy side dish that perfectly complements the chicken. Cranberry contains proanthocyanidins (PACs) that can prevent the adhesion of certain bacteria such as E. coli *to the urinary tract wall.*

Yield: 4 to 6 servings

Chicken:

1 teaspoon ground cinnamon
1 teaspoon ground cloves
1 teaspoon cayenne
1 teaspoon ground cumin
1 teaspoon fennel seeds
1 tablespoon sweet paprika
¾ teaspoon kosher salt
1 teaspoon brown sugar
Juice of ½ lemon
2 tablespoons olive oil
4 cloves garlic, crushed
1½ to 2 pounds boneless, skinless chicken breasts

Couscous:

1 cup couscous
10 dried apricots
½ cup dried cranberries
1½ cups boiling water
2 green onions, green parts only, chopped
2 handfuls of chopped fresh cilantro
Juice of ½ lemon
2 tablespoons extra-virgin olive oil
Kosher salt and freshly ground pepper

To make the chicken, combine all ingredients except the chicken in a large bowl and mix well to make a rich marinade. Add the chicken and let it marinate for at least 30 minutes— longer does make it taste better. While the chicken marinates, work on the couscous.

To make the couscous, put the couscous, apricots, and cranberries in a medium-size bowl and pour the boiling water over them, stirring with a fork to combine. Cover and let sit for 10 to 15 minutes, then uncover and fluff with a fork. Add the green onions and cilantro and drizzle with the lemon juice and olive oil. Season with the salt and pepper to taste and toss gently to combine. Set aside and keep warm.

Moroccan Chicken over Apricot-Cranberry Couscous (continued)

Red Hot Ingredient:
Apricots

• Vitamin A, C, and E
• Beta-carotene
• Lycopene

To make the dish, heat a skillet or grill pan over medium heat and add the chicken. Brown the chicken on both sides, watching carefully as the spice mixture on the chicken can make it burn rather easily After browning both sides, turn the heat down to low and put a lid over the skillet, this will allow the chicken to almost steam, making for a very moist chicken breast. When the chicken is fully cooked, remove it from the heat and let it rest for 10 minutes, then slice against the grain. Serve with the couscous.

—Joanne Choi

Per serving (chicken): 238 Cal.; 51 GI; 31 g Prot.; 4 g Carb.; 2 g SFA; 6 g MUFA; 2 g PUFA; 0.1 g Omega-3; 40 mg Calc.; 434 mg Sod.; 320 mg Pot.; 2 mg Iron; 0 mg Phytoestrogen; 1 g Fiber

Per serving (couscous): 252 Cal.; 55 GI; 6 g Prot.; 46 g Carb.; 0.8 g SFA; 4 g MUFA; 0.7 g PUFA; 0 g Omega-3; 25 mg Calc.; 10 mg Sod.; 262 mg Pot.; 1 mg Iron; 0 mg Phytoestrogen; 4 g Fiber

Roasted Chicken Mediterranean

This dish combines the flavors of Greece, Italy, and the South of France.

A beautiful and robust dish, it is easy to prepare and perfect for a dinner party. You may simplify it or embellish it in many ways. Some delicious additions include artichokes, oven-cured tomatoes, and grilled Swiss chard. Chicken on the bone adds flavor, but you may choose to use boneless breast instead. For less salt, use reduced-sodium chicken broth.

Yield: 4 servings

4 large, bone-in chicken breasts

Kosher salt

Cracked peppercorns

Pinch of dried oregano

I bay leaf

2 sprigs of fresh thyme

I bunch of fresh Italian (flat-leaf) parsley, chopped

I cup olive oil

3 lemons

4 Idaho potatoes, unpeeled

2 cloves garlic, halved

½ cup dry white wine

3 ounces sun-dried tomatoes

35 to 40 pitted kalamata olives

2 sprigs of fresh basil, sliced thinly

½ cup chicken broth

Place the chicken in a deep dish or bowl and season with the salt, cracked peppercorns, oregano, bay leaf, thyme, and half the chopped parsley. Pour ½ cup of the olive oil over the top. Roll the lemons on the countertop back and forth to "loosen up" all the juices. Cut one of the lemons in half and squeeze all the juice onto the chicken, then cut up a second lemon and add it to the bowl. Toss to mix well and coat the chicken. Marinate in the refrigerator for a couple of hours.

Wash the potatoes, dry them well, and cut each of them lengthwise into eight wedges. Heat a few teaspoons of the remaining ½ cup of olive oil in a skillet over high heat. Add the potatoes and sauté until browned on all sides. Set aside.

Roasted Chicken Mediterranean (continued)

Preheat the oven to 350°F.

Remove the chicken from the marinade and place in a heavy skillet. Brown thoroughly over medium-high heat. Transfer the chicken to a heavy roasting pan large enough to hold the chicken and potatoes. Place the garlic and browned potatoes around the chicken and bake for about 20 minutes, or until the chicken is tender and tests done with a meat thermometer.

Place the chicken and potatoes on a serving platter. Place the roasting pan on the stove over medium heat, add the wine, and bring to a boil to deglaze the pan. Add the sun-dried tomatoes, olives, basil, and the remaining olive oil and mix well. Add the chicken broth, the juice of the remaining lemon, and the rest of the parsley and bring to a boil again. Season to taste and spoon over the chicken and serve.

—*Carrie Nahabedian*

Per serving: 716 Cal.; 55 GI; 35 g Prot.; 59 g Carb.; 6 g SFA; 26 g MUFA; 5 g PUFA; 0.4 g Omega-3; 191 mg Calc.; 1,068 mg Sod.; 2,254 mg Pot.; 10 mg Iron; 0.012 mg Phytoestrogen; 11 g Fiber

Whole Roasted Baby Chicken and Potato Gnocchi with Honey-Glazed Parsnips and Young Beets

This recipe makes a truly tantalizing meal. Parsnips should really be part of everyone's diet. Looking to lose weight? Opt for parsnips over carrots—they provide double the fiber, which can fend off hunger pangs if you're trying to lose weight, plus they may lower cholesterol and keep blood sugar levels balanced. As a bonus, parsnips are a great source of vitamin K. For less saturated fat, substitute heart-healthy buttery spread for the butter.

Yield: 4 servings

Chicken:
4 whole poussins (baby chickens)
Salt and cracked peppercorns
A few sprigs of fresh thyme
¼ cup olive oil
4 teaspoons butter
½ cup dry white wine

Vegetables:
1 pound beets (golden, red, or Chioggia beets; baby or large)
2 tablespoons butter
2 parsnips, peeled and cut into preferred shape
2 tablespoons honey

Gnocchi:
2 tablespoons butter
16 potato gnocchi

Buy fresh baby chickens at a specialty butcher shop. Have the butcher truss them for you if possible. If not, chop the wing bones off at the center joint and trim the neck and skin. Truss by using kitchen string: start looping with the string around the feet, crossing down and over the wings and then to the neck. Knot and cut.

Season the chickens with salt and cracked peppercorns and stuff the insides with a few sprigs of thyme.

Preheat the oven to 350°F.

Heat the olive oil in a large skillet over medium-high heat. Pat the chickens dry and place them in the skillet and sauté until browned completely on all sides. Place the chickens in a roasting pan and dab a pat of butter on top of each bird. Place in the oven and roast for 25 minutes, or until a meat thermometer reaches 170°F. Remove from the oven, deglaze the pan with the wine, and reserve the roasting juices. Let the birds cool, and then

Whole Roasted Baby Chicken and Potato Gnocchi . . . (continued)

remove the meat from the bones. The meat can be refrigerated for 4 days for future use if desired.

To make the vegetables, place the beets in a saucepan filled with cold water and cook over medium-high heat until a knife can be easily inserted into the center of the beets. Cool under running cold water, then trim the beets and peel off their skins. Halve the beets or cut them into wedges, depending on the size. Set aside. The beets can be stored in the refrigerator for up to 4 days.

Preheat the oven to 350°F.

Heat the butter in a heavy ovenproof skillet over medium-high heat. Add the parsnips and sauté until tender. Drizzle the parsnips with the honey, place in the oven, and roast until they are glazed and caramelized. Set aside.

To prepare the gnocchi, heat the butter in a heavy skillet over medium-high heat. Add the gnocchi and sauté until cooked through. Set aside.

To serve, preheat the oven to 200°F. Place the chicken on a serving platter and place the gnocchi around the chicken. Top with the glazed parsnips and beets and place in the oven for a few minutes to heat through. Remove from the oven and drizzle with a good extra-virgin olive oil or with the pan juices from roasting the birds.

—Carrie Nahabedian

Per serving: 552 Cal.; 74 GI; 40 g Prot.; 69 g Carb.; 5 g SFA; 4 g MUFA; 2 g PUFA; 0.2 g Omega-3; 93 mg Calc.; 1,060 mg Sod.; 1,108 mg Pot.; 4 mg Iron; 0 mg Phyto-estrogen; 8 g Fiber

Grandma Greenwood's Roasted Sunday Chicken

Braising is a wonderful way to cook meats in the oven while you are at church or hanging out on a Sunday afternoon, because you don't need to worry about overcooking or burning your dinner. The result is a dish that is "fork tender," as chefs call it. Will Greenwood always loved Sundays, because when he and his family got home from church, they would always have a wonderful feast, which was part of their Southern heritage. They loved the "warmed-overs," too, as braised meats always reheat well and are, in fact, sometimes even better the next day. This dish is also a great way to get the kids to eat their vegetables, too—root vegetables are a great source of fiber, antioxidants, and vitamins. Note: If fresh herbs aren't available, substitute 1½ teaspoons of poultry seasoning.

Yield: 6 servings (plus leftovers)

1 (4½- to 5-pound) roasting chicken
2 pounds fingerling potatoes
1 pound peeled baby carrots
1 pound turnips, peeled and halved
1 pound rutabaga, peeled and cut into large dice
1 head cabbage, quartered and cored
1 pound parsnips, peeled and cut into large dice
1 pound pearl onions, peeled
2 heads garlic, halved crosswise to expose the individual cloves of garlic
2 sprigs of fresh thyme
2 sprigs of fresh oregano
2 sprigs of fresh rosemary
4 cups chicken broth
1 (2-ounce) envelope Lipton onion soup
All-purpose flour

Preheat the oven to 320°F.

Remove the inside pouch and neck from the chicken and reserve for another use. Wash the chicken well in cold water and pat dry. Place it in a large roasting pan and arrange the vegetables around the chicken. Add the herbs and set aside. (If using poultry seasoning instead of fresh herbs, add it in the next step.)

Pour the broth into a saucepan and place over medium heat. Add the onion soup powder and poultry seasoning (if using). Stir and cook until dissolved, and then pour the mixture into the roasting pan. Cover the pan, place it in the oven, and braise for 1½ to 2 hours, or until a leg easily pulls away from the joint.

Grandma Greenwood's Roasted Sunday Chicken (continued)

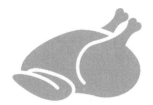

When done, remove from the oven and transfer the chicken to a large serving platter and arrange the vegetables around it. Pour the pan juices into a pitcher or fat separator, and when the fat rises to the top, pour the defatted juices into a saucepan and bring to a simmer on the stove. Add the flour, a little at a time, and stir until you have a sauce that is thickened to your taste. Pour the sauce into a gravy boat and serve on the side.

—Will Greenwood

Per serving: 789 Cal.; 72 GI; 55 g Prot.; 121 g Carb.; 3 g SFA; 4 g MUFA; 3 g PUFA; 0.4 g Omega-3; 417 mg Calc.; 1,332 mg Sod.; 3,580 mg Pot.; 9 mg Iron; 0 mg Phytoestrogen; 27 g Fiber

Delectable Sweet-and-Sour Tofu

If you think you don't like heart-healthy tofu, you probably just haven't had it prepared the right way! This dish is delicious served with rice and green beans.

Yield: 4 servings

I pound extra-firm tofu
I tablespoon vegetable or peanut oil

Sauce:
Juice and zest of I lime
¼ cup freshly squeezed orange juice
½ teaspoon lemon pepper seasoning
I tablespoon reduced-sodium soy sauce
I tablespoon Asian sweet chili sauce, or
    I tablespoon orange marmalade and
    ⅛ teaspoon red pepper flakes

Red Hot Ingredient:
Tofu

- Calcium, copper, iron, magnesium, and phosphorus
- Protein
- Omega-3 fatty acids
- Isoflavones
- Phytoestrogens

Variation:

Add ½ teaspoon of Asian Chili Garlic Sauce to the marinade.

Drain the tofu, wrap it in a clean dishcloth, and let it rest for at least 10 minutes and up to 2 hours to remove the water.

Cut the tofu crosswise into three equal rectangles, and then cut each rectangle into 4 long strips.

To make the sauce, in a mixing bowl, combine the lime juice and zest, orange juice, lemon pepper seasoning, soy sauce, and chili sauce and mix well. Set aside.

Heat the oil in a large nonstick skillet over medium to medium-high heat until the oil is very hot. Add the tofu strips in a single layer and let them cook for about 4 minutes on each side, until they are medium brown on the top and bottom.

When the tofu is browned, add the sauce and let it boil down for about 2 minutes, until the sauce is thick. Remove from the heat and serve immediately.

—Aviva Goldfarb

Per serving: 154 Cal.; 34 GI; 12 g Prot.; 7 g Carb.; 1 g SFA; 6 g MUFA; 2 g PUFA; 0.006 g Omega-3; 212 mg Calc.; 243 mg Sod.; 227 mg Pot.; 2 mg Iron; 26 mg Phytoestrogen; 2 g Fiber

Grilled Marinated Tempeh

Tempeh provides probiotics, the "good" bacteria that your body needs. It is also high in protein and a great substitute for milk and meat in your diet. Tempeh is also high in phytoestrogens, which help some women's hot flashes. So fire up the grill and see if this healthy meal can turn down your heat.

Yield: 4 servings

¼ cup lemon juice

¼ cup olive oil

¼ teaspoon dried thyme

Freshly ground pepper

16 ounces tempeh

1 large onion, sliced into rings

4 whole wheat hamburger rolls

Lettuce and tomato slices, for garnish (optional)

Red Hot Ingredient: Tempeh

• Vitamins A and B$_{12}$

• Calcium

• Fiber

• Phytoestrogens

To prepare the marinade, combine the lemon juice, olive oil, thyme, and pepper to taste in a small bowl; set aside. Cut the tempeh into four slices. Using a steamer, steam the tempeh for 15 minutes. Place the tempeh and onions in a 2-quart casserole and pour the marinade over them. Refrigerate for at least 4 hours.

Preheat the oven to 400°F.

Cover the casserole dish and bake for 30 to 35 minutes (or grill, basting frequently with the marinade). Serve hot on hamburger rolls, garnished with lettuce and tomato if desired.

—*Dr. Mache's Kitchen*

Per serving: 471 Cal.; 55 GI; 27 g Prot.; 35 g Carb.; 5 g SFA; 14 g MUFA; 6 g PUFA; 0.37 g Omega-3; 191 mg Calc.; 220 mg Sod.; 762 mg Pot.; 4 mg Iron; 50 mg Phytoestrogen; 8 g Fiber

Eggplant-Tofu No-Noodle Lasagne

This is a wonderful vegetarian lasagne that uses eggplant instead of pasta. It's easy to make and delicious. Choose eggplants that are shiny with wrinkle-free skin. They should feel springy, not spongy. You'll reap the health benefits from their chlorogenic acid, a phenol antioxidant that scavenges disease-causing free radicals. Enjoy!

Yield: 4 servings

1 tablespoon olive oil or oil spray

1 large eggplant, peeled and cut into ¼-inch strips

3 cups pasta sauce (store-bought or homemade)

1 (1-pound) brick extra-firm tofu, sliced

4 tomatoes, sliced

1 bunch of fresh basil, leaves separated

1 (1-pound) package shredded mozzarella cheese

½ pound grated Parmesan cheese

Preheat the oven to 350°F. Grease a cookie sheet and an 8-inch square baking dish with the olive oil or cooking spray.

Place the eggplant strips on the greased cookie sheet and bake for 10 minutes, or until tender. Set aside.

Spoon ¾ cup of the pasta sauce into the greased baking dish and place one-third of the eggplant strips (in place of noodles) as the first layer of the lasagne. Add one-third of the tofu slices in another layer, followed by one-third of the sliced tomatoes and then one-third of the basil leaves. Spoon another ¾ cup of the pasta sauce over the basil, followed by one-third of the mozzarella and Parmesan cheeses. Repeat the same layers twice more, ending with a layer of pasta sauce topped with the cheeses. Place in the oven and bake for 45 minutes. Serve immediately.

—Catherine D'Amato

Per serving: 542 Cal.; 50 GI; 43 g Prot.; 35 g Carb.; 12 g SFA; 12 g MUFA; 1 g PUFA; 0.2 g Omega-3; 1,071 mg Calc.; 1,333 mg Sod.; 1,176 mg Pot.; 5 mg Iron; 34 mg Phytoestrogen; 9 g Fiber

Charcoal-Grilled Seitan Skewers

This recipe is known as "Seitan Chimichurris" at the Candle Café and Candle 79 restaurant in New York City, where it is one of the restaurant's all-time favorites. They have been known to ship these appetizers to friends and customers on the West Coast who have called in need of a fix. These seitan skewers freeze very well and are great to have on hand to serve as a healthy appetizer, snack, or entrée. The protein in seitan is similar to that in beef (26 grams per ½ cup), but it's all made from wheat. It's a great meat substitute.

Yield: 6 servings (2 skewers each)

1 cup freshly squeezed lemon juice

1 cup olive oil

2 cloves garlic, minced

¼ cup agave syrup

1 teaspoon salt

½ cup finely chopped fresh Italian (flat-leaf) parsley

1 cup finely chopped fresh cilantro

1½ pounds seitan, cut into 1½-inch pieces

Per serving (about 2 tablespoons) (marinade): 169 Cal.; 30 GI; 0.2 g Prot.; 2 g Carb.; 2 g SFA; 13 g MUFA; 2 g PUFA; 0.1 g Omega-3; 19 mg Calc.; 199 mg Sod.; 50 mg Pot.; 0.5 mg Iron; 0 mg Phytoestrogen; 0.5 g Fiber

Per serving (seitan skewers): 518 Cal.; 69 GI; 104 g Prot.; 20 g Carb.; 0.3 g SFA; 0.2 g MUFA; 1 g PUFA; 0.06 g Omega-3; 201 mg Calc.; 386 mg Sod.; 156 mg Pot.; 7 mg Iron; 0.05 mg Phytoestrogen; 1 g Fiber

To prepare the marinade, put the lemon juice, olive oil, garlic, agave syrup, salt, parsley, and cilantro in a food processor and blend on high speed until well combined.

To prepare the seitan skewers, put four pieces of seitan on each of twelve metal skewers and place them in a large, nonreactive bowl or baking dish. Pour the marinade over them and let them marinate for at least 1 hour or overnight.

Prepare a charcoal, gas, or stove-top grill. Remove the seitan skewers from the marinade and pour the marinade into a sauceboat. Grill the skewers over medium-high heat until well browned, 5 to 7 minutes per side. Serve immediately with the marinade on the side.

—*Benay Vynerib*

Tofu Cacciatore

This spicy vegetarian dish is chock-full of great nutrients such as protein, phytoestrogens, calcium, and fiber. If hot flashes are on your mind, go easy on the Cajun seasoning.

Yield: 8 to 10 servings

Cajun Seasoning:
4 tablespoons chili powder
3 tablespoons paprika
1½ tablespoons garlic powder
1 tablespoon kosher salt
1 tablespoon freshly ground pepper

Cacciatore:
Olive oil
8 cloves garlic, minced
Kosher salt
Freshly ground pepper
2 Vidalia onions, chopped
2 green bell peppers, seeded and chopped
1 red bell pepper, seeded and chopped
Italian seasoning
2 pounds organic firm tofu, cut into ½-inch sheets
Cajun seasoning (above)
A couple of splashes of dry red wine
Dash of Worcestershire sauce (optional)
1 (26-ounce) jar tomato-basil sauce
¼ to ½ cup spicy red pepper sauce
½ pound feta cheese
Grated Parmesan cheese and/or Romano and Asiago cheeses
Pinch of paprika
2 (1-pound) packages pasta
1 cup chopped fresh Italian (flat-leaf) parsley

To make the Cajun seasoning, combine all the seasoning ingredients in small bowl and mix well. Set aside.

To make the cacciatore, heat a generous amount of olive oil in a large saucepan over medium-high heat. Add the garlic and sauté for 1 minute. Add a shake of kosher salt and pepper and the onions and sauté for another 1 to 2 minutes, then add the bell peppers and some Italian seasoning and sauté for a few more minutes. Remove from the heat and spoon into a large casserole, leaving whatever olive oil is left in the saucepan.

Preheat the oven to 375°F.

Add more olive oil to the saucepan and put it back on the stove over medium-high heat. Coat the tofu sheets with the Cajun seasoning and fry them for a few minutes on each side until they are crispy. As the tofu is fried, add it to the casserole with the onion mixture and toss the onion mixture over the tofu. Splash with the wine and the Worcestershire sauce if using. Cover with the tomato-basil

Tofu Cacciatore (continued)

and spicy red pepper sauces and place over medium heat. When it begins to bubble, use a sturdy spatula to lift up the tofu so the mixture can get underneath. Lower the heat to medium and crumble the feta cheese over the top. Liberally sprinkle with the Parmesan cheese, and then with a little Italian seasoning, finishing with a shake or two of paprika. Bake in the oven for 35 to 40 minutes, until bubbling and slightly crispy brown.

Cook the pasta al dente according to the package instructions. Drain, return to the saucepan, and cover with a little olive oil, Parmesan cheese, and the chopped parsley. Serve the tofu cacciatore over the pasta, with a loaf of crusty bread if you like.

—*Ben Schwendener*

Per serving: 665 Cal.; 44 GI; 36 g Prot.; 79 g Carb.; 6 g SFA; 16 g MUFA; 3 g PUFA; 0.2 g Omega-3; 543 mg Calc.; 612 mg Sod.; 827 mg Pot.; 8 mg Iron; 47 mg Phytoestrogen; 11 g Fiber

Cold Tofu with Cilantro, Green Onions, and Soy Sesame Sauce

This simple, nutritious tofu dish is a deliciously healthy meat substitute for lunch or dinner. And the phytoestrogens make it a great dish for hot flashes and building strong bones.

Yield: 4 to 6 servings

1 (1-pound) package soft (silken) tofu
1 tablespoon soy sauce
1 tablespoon sesame oil
3 tablespoons chopped green onions
2 tablespoons chopped fresh cilantro

Carefully slice the tofu into equal-size pieces (about ½ inch thick). Lay them flat on a plate.

In a small bowl, combine the soy sauce and sesame oil and drizzle a little over the top of each tofu slice. Then sprinkle the tofu with the green onions and cilantro and serve.

—Joanne Choi

Per serving: 83 Cal.;19 GI; 6.5 g Prot.; 3 g Carb.; 1 g SFA; 2 g MUFA; 2 g PUFA; 0.1 g Omega-3; 32 mg Calc.; 213 mg Sod.; 194 mg Pot.; 1 mg Iron; 26 mg Phytoestrogen; 0 g Fiber

Byaldi Confit and Crispy Artichokes with Saffron-Tomato Nage

A spin on the traditional ratatouille, this recipe is hearty for body and soul. The French are able to stay so slender because they eat healthy dishes with lots of vegetables and salad. This is a great recipe to sneak more vegetables into your diet. Use any vegetables you like, but this recipe uses a combination of zucchini, eggplant, summer squash, tomato, and artichoke that has just the right texture. It is a perfect example of fresh, low-fat and healthy cuisine.

Yield: 10 servings

Byaldi Confit:
3 tablespoons olive oil, plus more for seasoning

3 red onions, sliced thinly

Salt and pepper

4 zucchini, sliced into ⅛-inch-thick rounds

4 Japanese eggplants, sliced into 1/8-inch-thick rounds

4 yellow summer squash, sliced into ⅛-inch-thick rounds

5 Roma tomatoes, sliced into ⅛-inch-thick rounds

Crispy Artichokes:
3 large artichokes, stripped of leaves, choked, and soaked in lemon water

Salt

4 cups or more olive oil

¼ teaspoon dried thyme

Saffron-Tomato Nage:
2 tablespoons olive oil

1 white onion, chopped

2 cloves garlic, chopped

2 shallots, chopped

4 Roma tomatoes, chopped

Pinch of saffron

½ cup white wine

2 cups vegetable broth or water

4 tablespoons butter (½ stick)

To make the byaldi confit, preheat the oven to 275°F. Heat the 3 tablespoons of olive oil in a skillet over medium heat. Add the onions and cook slowly, stirring occasionally, until caramelized. Season with salt and pepper and spread evenly on a rimmed baking sheet. Arrange alternating slices of the vegetables— one slice each of zucchini, eggplant, squash,

Continues ...

Byaldi Confit and Crispy Artichokes with Saffron-Tomato Nabe (continued)

and tomato—in rows over the onions, overlapping so that ¼ inch of each slice is exposed. Season with salt and olive oil and cover with foil. Bake in the oven for 2 hours. Remove from the oven, take off the foil, and set aside.

To make the artichokes, preheat the oven to 300°F. Drain the artichokes, place them in a baking dish, and season them with salt. Pour enough olive oil over the artichokes to submerge them, then stir in the thyme. Cover and bake for 45 minutes, or until fork tender. When cooked, remove the artichokes from the baking dish and let drain on paper towels. (Reserve a few teaspoons of the olive oil.) When cool enough to handle, slice the artichokes thinly. Heat the reserved olive oil in a skillet over high heat, add the artichoke slices, and fry until golden brown. Set aside.

To make the saffron-tomato nage, heat the olive oil in a saucepan over medium-high heat. Add the onion, garlic, and shallots and sauté until the vegetables are tender. Add the tomatoes, saffron, wine, and broth and bring to a simmer. Cook uncovered until the sauce has reduced by one-third. Stir in the butter and strain through a chinois strainer into a sauceboat.

To serve, preheat the broiler, place the byaldi confit underneath, and broil until the vegetables are lightly browned. Serve the byaldi confit and the crispy artichokes with the nage on the side.

—*Chef Neal Fraser*

Per serving: 201 Cal.; 60 GI; 6 g Prot.; 28 g Carb.; 3 g SFA; 4 g MUFA; 1 g PUFA; 0.1 g Omega-3; 70 mg Calc.; 391 mg Sod.; 1,194 mg Pot.; 2 mg Iron; 0 mg Phyto-estrogen; 12 g Fiber

Oven-Roasted Artichokes with Garlic and Anchovies

Artichokes are one of the most antioxidant-dense vegetables. Many experts believe that the unwanted effects of aging is caused by the degenerative effects of free radicals, which can be reduced if enough antioxidants are consumed. Serve alone as a main course, or as an appetizer.

Yield: 4 servings

4 large artichokes

Juice of ¼ lemon

Salt

2 teaspoons anchovy paste, or 4 small fillets, scraped and minced

2 shallots, minced

4 cloves garlic, minced

I cup fresh bread crumbs or panko

3 tablespoons chopped fresh Italian (flat-leaf) parsley

4 tablespoons olive oil

I lemon, cut into 4 wedges

Preheat the oven to 375°F.

Trim the stems from the bottom of the artichokes so that they will sit up on a plate. Reserve the stems. Bring 2 to 3 quarts of water to a boil in a large saucepan. Add the artichokes, their stems, the lemon juice, and 1 teaspoon of salt and cook at a rolling boil for 8 to 10 minutes, or until they are three-quarters cooked. Take the artichokes and stems out of the water with a slotted spoon and let them drain and cool on a cookie sheet.

When the artichokes are cool enough to handle, spread the leaves out and remove and discard the inner leaves. Using a small teaspoon, scrape out the inner chokes and discard them. Set the artichokes aside. Cut the stems up into a small dice and place them in a small bowl. Add the anchovy paste, a pinch of salt,

Continues . . .

Oven-Roasted Artichokes with Garlic and Anchovies (continued)

and the shallot, garlic, bread crumbs, parsley, and salt and pepper to taste to the bowl and toss lightly to combine. Place the artichokes in a shallow baking dish so they sit with their leaves facing up. Lightly fill the cavity of each with 2 to 3 tablespoons of the bread crumb filling. Spread out the leaves slightly and sprinkle the remaining filling between the leaves.

Drizzle each artichoke with 1 tablespoon of olive oil and a few drops of lemon juice. Fill the bottom of the baking dish with ¼ inch of water.

Place the artichokes in the oven and bake for 20 to 30 minutes, or until the artichokes are warm and the bread crumbs are golden brown and toasted on the top. Serve hot from the oven as a main dish with lemon wedges on the side.

—Gordon Hamersley

Per serving: 320 Cal.; 65 GI; 8 g Prot.; 40 g Carb.; 2 g SFA; 10 g MUFA; 2 g PUFA; 0.2 g Omega-3; 96 mg Calc.; 1,054 mg Sod.; 523 mg Pot.; 3 mg Iron; 0.3 mg Phytoestrogen; 12 g Fiber

---

Do You Remember When Your Mother Used to Say . . .

"Eat your vegetables, they're good, and they're good for you"? She was right! To stay well, eat a lot of them; more as you grow older. If you're physically active, you may be able to eat even more and not gain weight. Eating vegetables daily helps prevent certain diseases, including some cancers, and helps control your weight.

Meatless Sloppy Joes

Enjoy this healthy approach to an American classic. It's easy to make and good for you. Vegetable protein can be used as a substitute for many meat dishes. This recipe is so full of phytoestrogens, calcium, and almost no saturated fat, you won't miss the meat.

Yield: 4 servings

I cup textured vegetable protein (TVP)
I cup boiling water
I (16-ounce) can Sloppy Joe sauce
4 whole wheat hamburger rolls

Place the textured vegetable protein in a medium-size saucepan and pour the boiling water over it to rehydrate. Stir and let stand for 5 to 10 minutes. Stir in the Sloppy Joe sauce and cook over medium heat for 3 to 4 minutes, or until thoroughly heated. Spoon the mixture onto four buns and serve.

—Dr. Mache's Kitchen

Per serving: 298 Cal.; 74 GI; 19 g Prot.; 46 g Carb.; 1 g SFA; 2 g MUFA; 2 g PUFA; 0.15 g Omega-3; 137 mg Calc.; 766 mg Sod.; 1,062 mg Pot.; 5 mg Iron; 37 mg Phytoestrogen; 8 g Fiber

Savor Your Food

Eat slowly and experience your food; put your fork down between bites; avoid eating while watching TV; and don't jump up immediately from the table when finished eating—relax a moment and digest!

Baked Eggplant

Eggplant is a very healthy vegetable. This recipe makes a wonderful vegetarian meal straight from Bubbie's Kitchen.

Yield: 4 servings

2 medium-size eggplants, peeled and cut into 2-inch chunks

3 cups boiling water

Salt

2 tablespoons vegetable oil

2 medium-size onions, chopped

1 clove garlic, minced

1 large egg, beaten

¼ cup bread crumbs

Freshly ground pepper

Preheat the oven to 350°F.

Place the eggplant chunks in a saucepan with the boiling water and a pinch of salt and boil for 5 to 10 minutes, or until tender. Drain and set aside.

Heat the oil in a saucepan over medium-high heat. Add the onions and garlic and sauté until golden brown. Add the eggplant, egg, and bread crumbs and season with salt and pepper. Transfer the eggplant mixture to an 8-inch square baking pan and bake for 15 to 20 minutes, until browned. (You can sprinkle some bread crumbs over the top before baking if you wish.)

—*Bubbie's Kitchen*

Per serving: 198 Cal.; 61 GI; 6 g Prot.; 26 g Carb.; 1 g SFA; 5 g MUFA; 2 g PUFA; 0.6 g Omega-3; 64 mg Calc.; 375 mg Sod.; 770 mg Pot.; 1 mg Iron; 0.073 mg Phytoestrogen; 11 g Fiber

Lemon- and Mint-Marinated Roast Leg of Lamb

Roasted lamb is the typical meat choice for spring dinners, and this roast lamb dish is exceptionally delicious. Lamb is also rich in selenium, which can help ward off asthma attacks. All will enjoy the sweet, rich flavor of this dish. Note: The tomatoes and garlic confit can be prepared ahead of time.

Yield: 8 to 12 servings

Tomatoes:

12 Roma tomatoes, cored and halved lengthwise

Salt and pepper

1 cup olive oil

3 sprigs of fresh thyme

Garlic Confit:

4 heads garlic, cloves separated and peeled

1 cup olive oil, plus more for drizzling

Flageolets:

1 (4-ounce) slab bacon, sliced and then cut into ¼-inch pieces (optional)

1 medium-size onion, finely chopped

1 sprig of fresh thyme

1 bunch of fresh parsley

1 bay leaf

2 pounds flageolet beans, rinsed and drained

4 cups chicken broth, fresh or canned

Lamb:

1 semiboneless leg of lamb (inner thigh bone removed and leg tied with twine)

Kosher salt and cracked peppercorns

Olive oil

2 bunches of fresh mint, torn

2 lemons

75 pitted kalamata olives, rinsed and halved lengthwise

To prepare the tomatoes, preheat the oven to 400°F, leave on for 2 hours, and then turn the heat off.

Place the tomatoes, cut side up, on the rack of a baking pan. Season generously with salt and pepper. Drizzle the tomatoes with the olive oil and add the sprigs of thyme. Place the tomatoes in the oven overnight to cure and dry. Remove the tomatoes from the oven in the morning. They should be slightly caramelized and semidry, but still plump. If the desired effect is not achieved overnight, you can turn the oven back on and dry the tomatoes out for no more than 30 minutes. The tomatoes can be prepared up to 3 days in advance and kept in the refrigerator.

Continues ...

Lemon- and Mint-Marinated Roast Leg of Lamb (continued)

To make the garlic confit, preheat the oven to 325°F.

Set aside eight cloves of the garlic. Place the remaining cloves in a baking dish and cover with 1 cup of olive oil. Bake until the garlic cloves are soft but still firm enough to keep their shape. Remove from the oven and let cool in the oil. This can be done up to a week in advance and the garlic can be stored in the refrigerator.

To make the flageolets, preheat the oven to 350°F.

Place the bacon (if using) in a heavy casserole or deep 3-quart saucepan and cook over high heat to render the bacon fat. (If not using the bacon, heat 3 tablespoons of olive oil instead.) Add the onions and sauté until tender. Add four of the uncooked garlic cloves, the sprig of thyme, the parsley, and the bay leaf. Stir in the flageolets and coat them thoroughly. Add a nice drizzle of olive oil, and then pour in the chicken broth to cover the flageolets. Bring to a boil and then place in the oven covered with either buttered parchment paper or a lid. Cook very slowly and carefully for about 1 hour, until the flageolets are firm but tender and cooked through. Do not overcook! Check the flageolets at least twice during cooking and stir them gently. Remove from the oven and let cool in their juice. (The juice will become the sauce.)

To make the lamb, preheat the oven to 375°F. With a sharp knife, remove and discard the thick excess of fat from the lamb. Season with the kosher salt and cracked peppercorns, and then rub it with olive oil. Mince two of the uncooked garlic cloves and place the leg of lamb in a heavy roasting pan and rub it with half the torn mint and the minced garlic. Thinly slice the remaining two cloves of uncooked garlic. With the tip of a paring knife, gently jab the lamb in various spots and place a sliver of garlic in each slit. This adds an added boost of flavor!

Roll the lemons on your countertop (this produces the maximum juice), then cut them in half and squeeze the juice over the top of the lamb and rub it in. Place in the oven and roast to your desired doneness. Medium-rare to medium will take about 90 minutes. Baste the lamb many times during roasting to add flavor and moistness.

Lemon- and Mint-Marinated Roast Leg of Lamb (continued)

To serve, place the lamb on a cutting board and let rest for 10 minutes. Slice the lamb and place on a serving platter or individual plates. Place the oven-cured tomatoes around the lamb and sprinkle with the olives. With a slotted spoon, spoon the flageolets over the meat. Heat the juice quickly over medium-high heat, add the remaining torn mint and infuse for a couple of minutes. Spoon the garlic confit over the flageolets and then drizzle with the pan juices from the lamb.

The leg will serve eight very generously and the remainder makes a great meal the next day.

—*Carrie Nahabedian*

Per serving: 918 Cal.; 32 GI; 46 g Prot.; 59 g Carb.; 7 g SFA; 39 g MUFA; 6 g PUFA; 0.8 g Omega-3; 169 mg Calc.; 687 mg Sod.; 1,485 mg Pot.; 10 mg Iron; 0.89 mg Phytoestrogen; 17 g Fiber

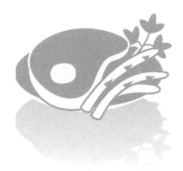

12

DESSERTS

Apples with Raisins

This is a homey dessert that's easy to make and difficult to resist. We've all heard "an apple a day keeps the doctor away"; it's all because of the health benefits of apples. Eating apples, which uniquely contain phloridzin, a flavanoid that may be help build strong bones, may protect women from osteoporosis, increase bone density, and help lower risk of developing certain cancers. If you wish, substitute a heart-healthy buttery spread for the butter.

Yield: 4 servings

¼ cup golden raisins

1 teaspoon ground cinnamon

½ teaspoon ground ginger

Pinch of ground cumin

2 tablespoons butter

4 apples

5 tablespoons muscat dessert wine

Preheat the oven to 325°F. Lightly grease a baking dish with a small amount of butter.

Soak the raisins in hot water for about 10 minutes to rehydrate. Drain the raisins, and then combine them in a small bowl with the cinnamon, ginger, and cumin. Set aside.

Core the apples, fill each cavity with the raisin mixture, and place the apples in the greased baking dish. Dot the apples with the butter, sprinkle with the wine, and bake for 30 minutes. Remove from the oven and let cool slightly before serving.

—Karen's Cucina

Per serving: 205 Cal.; 46 GI; 1 g Prot.; 35 g Carb.; 4 g SFA; 1 g MUFA; 0 g PUFA; 0.04 g Omega-3; 27 mg Calc.; 46 mg Sod.; 289 mg Pot.; 0.5 mg Iron; 0.032 mg Phytoestrogen; 5 g Fiber

Stuffed Pears

This special dessert is easy to make and absolutely delicious, and it is healthy and low in fat. The wine combined with the sweetness of the high-fiber pears makes a scrumptious dish. Almonds are a rich source of vitamin E, may lower LDL (bad) cholesterol, and may prevent certain cancers.

Yield: 4 servings

½ cup sliced almonds, toasted and chopped finely

1 tablespoon confectioners' sugar

2 large ripe pears, halved and cored

3 tablespoons dry Marsala wine

Red Hot Ingredient: Pears

- Vitamins B$_2$, C, and E
- Copper and potassium
- Pectin
- Fiber

Preheat the oven to 400°F. Lightly grease a baking dish with a small amount of butter.

Combine the almonds and sugar in a small bowl and mix well.

Place each pear half in the greased baking dish so that they fit snugly together. Stuff each pear half with the nut mixture, and then pour a little of the Marsala on top of each pear. Bake uncovered for 10 minutes. Serve warm.

—*Karen's Cucina*

Per serving: 190 Cal.; 37 GI; 4 g Prot.; 24 g Carb.; 1 g SFA; 5 g MUFA; 2 g PUFA; 0 g Omega-3; 59 mg Calc.; 2 mg Sod.; 261 mg Pot.; 1 mg Iron; 0 mg Phytoestrogen; 5 g Fiber

Strawberries with Ricotta Topping

Strawberries have high amounts of antioxidants, which may reduce our risk for developing cancer, cardiovascular disease, and inflammation-related diseases. They are filled with unusual phytonutrients that promote good health. Calcium-rich ricotta cheese, used in many Italian desserts, also offers many health benefits.

Yield: 4 servings

¼ cup coarsely chopped walnuts

¼ cup white chocolate chunks

1 (15-ounce) package nonfat ricotta cheese, crumbled

1 (4-ounce) package light cream cheese

¼ cup sugar

2 tablespoons vanilla extract

Fresh strawberries

Place the walnuts and chocolate in a food processor and pulse until the mixture becomes coarse in texture. Place the cheeses, sugar, and vanilla in a medium-size mixing bowl and mix well to combine. Refrigerate until ready to serve. Cut the strawberries in half and place them in individual serving bowls. Place a few spoonfuls of the cheese mixture on top of the strawberries, sprinkle with the walnut mixture, and serve.

—Karen's Cucina

Per serving: 363 Cal.; 48 GI; 21 g Prot.; 41 g Carb.; 5 g SFA; 3 g MUFA; 4 g PUFA; 1 g Omega-3; 286 mg Calc.; 233 mg Sod.; 592 mg Pot.; 1 mg Iron; 0 mg Phytoestrogen; 4 g Fiber

Red Hot Ingredient: Ricotta Cheese

- Vitamins A, B_1, B_2, and E, niacin, and folic acid
- Calcium, phosphorous, selenium, and zinc
- Protein

What happens to your weight when you eat too much candy? It goes up, right? That's because candy has a lot of sugar and almost no nutrients that your body needs to stay healthy and strong. Want an easy way to lose weight? Stop drinking soda and other sweetened drinks.

Peaches in Wine

Peaches in red wine are a great simple summer dessert after you've enjoyed a fabulous meal. Peaches contain a high amount of dietary fiber needed for good digestion; as well as carotenoids, which help eyes, and antioxidants that may protect against certain cancers.

Yield: 4 servings

6 ripe yellow peaches

1 cup Chianti wine

½ cup sugar

1 teaspoon ground cinnamon

½ teaspoon ground cloves

4 sprigs of fresh mint

In a large saucepan, bring 2 quarts of water to a boil. Add the peaches and boil for 15 seconds, and then remove them from the heat and let cool. When cool enough to handle, peel off the skins and remove the pits. Then cut the peaches into ¼-inch slices and set aside.

Put the wine, sugar, cinnamon, and cloves in a medium-size saucepan and cook over medium heat for 10 minutes, until reduced to a light syrup. Remove from the heat and let cool.

Place the sliced peaches in four wineglasses, then pour the syrup over them and garnish with the sprigs of mint. Serve immediately.

—*Karen's Cucina*

Per serving: 237 Cal.; 48 GI; 2 g Prot.; 49 g Carb.; 0 g SFA; 0.1 g MUFA; 0.2 g PUFA; 0 g Omega-3; 27 mg Calc.; 3 mg Sod.; 509 mg Pot.; 1 mg Iron; 0 mg Phytoestrogen; 4 g Fiber

Honey-Poached Pears with Citrus Biscotti

Enjoy this delicious dessert for the perfect end to your favorite meal. Enjoy it in small portions, as it tends to have a high calorie content but tastes truly divine.

Yield: 6 servings

Biscotti:
2¾ cups whole wheat flour
1⅔ cups sugar
1 teaspoon baking powder
½ teaspoon kosher salt
1 large egg
3 large egg yolks
2 teaspoons vanilla extract
2 tablespoons zest (lemon, lime, or orange)

Pears:
1½ cups honey
1½ cups dry white wine
1 tablespoon lemon juice
6 Bartlett pears, peeled and halved

To make the biscotti, preheat the oven to 350°F. Line a baking sheet with parchment paper.

Put the flour, sugar, baking powder, and salt into the bowl of a food processor.

In a mixing bowl, whisk together the whole egg, egg yolks, and vanilla and add to the dry ingredients in the processor. Mix on low speed, stopping to scrape the bowl occasionally. Add the zest and mix to combine, and then turn out the batter onto a floured work surface and shape it into a long, flattish log.

Place the log on the prepared baking sheet pan and bake the biscotti for 5 to 10 minutes, until it is a light golden color and feels firm to the touch. Let cool for 45 minutes.

Preheat the oven to 300°F. Cut the biscotti into ¼-inch slices and lay them on their side on the baking sheet. Bake for about 15 minutes, or until they begin to dry. Remove from the oven to let cool slightly, then test for crispness. If necessary, return the biscotti to the oven for a few more minutes until they are crisp. Let cool completely and store in an airtight container or sealable plastic bags.

To make the pears, place the honey, wine, lemon juice, and 1 cup of water in a nonreactive saucepan and bring to a boil over medium-high heat. Add the pears, lower the heat to a simmer, and poach the pears until tender, about 8 minutes and up to 25 minutes, depending on how ripe the pears are. When tender, remove from the heat and let cool in the poaching liquid.

When cool, remove the pears with a slotted spoon from the poaching liquid and set aside. Place the saucepan over medium-high heat and cook the poaching liquid until it is reduced to a syrup. Remove from the heat and set aside at room temperature.

To serve, place two pear halves in each of six individual serving dishes. Top with some of the syrup, and serve with the biscotti on the side.

—*Gordon Hamersley and Kristin Wilson*

Per serving: 608 Cal.; 66 GI; 11 g Prot.; 140 g Carb.; 1 g SFA; 1 g MUFA; 1 g PUFA; 0 g Omega-3; 107 mg Calc.; 629 mg Sod.; 559 mg Pot.; 3 mg Iron; 0 mg Phytoestrogen; 12 g Fiber

Baked Apples

This is a very simple and fast recipe that will impress the book club or whomever you have over. It really tastes delicious, is low in calories, and is the perfect ending to any meal. It's one of my favorite desserts.

Yield: 4 servings

4 Rome or Cortland apples

¼ cup raisins, dried cranberries, or dried cherries

¼ cup chopped walnuts

½ cup orange juice

Preheat the oven to 350°F.

Core the apples and place upright in a medium-size Pyrex baking dish. Combine the raisins and walnuts and fill each cavity with the mixture. Pour 2 tablespoons of the orange juice into each of the openings. Place in the oven and bake for 45 minutes, or until the apples are easily pierced with the tip of a knife. Cool and serve.

—Dr. Mache's Kitchen

Per serving: 185 Cal.; 45 GI; 2 g Prot.; 36 g Carb.; 0.5 g SFA; 1 g MUFA; 3 g PUFA; 1 g Omega-3; 27 mg Calc.; 4 mg Sod.; 353 mg Pot.; 1 mg Iron; 0 mg Phytoestrogen; 5 g Fiber

Variations:

- Refrigerate and serve cold.
- Sprinkle with cinnamon before serving.
- Garnish with a dollop of non-fat whipped cream.

Baked Spiced Pears with Zabaglione Sauce

Pears with cinnamon and cardamom are a marriage made in culinary heaven, says
Good Carbs, Bad Carbs *author Johanna Burani. This full-bodied dessert relies exclusively*
on the wholesome flavors of its ingredients and not added fats, making it an excellent
finish to a hearty holiday meal—or even Christmas dinner.

Yield: 4 servings

2 ripe Bosc pears
1 tablespoon LoGiCane sugar
¼ teaspoon ground cinnamon
¼ teaspoon ground cardamom

Sauce:

1 egg yolk
1 tablespoon LoGiCane sugar
2 tablespoons Marsala wine

*—University of Sydney Glycemic Index
and GI Database*

Per serving: 99 Cal.; 44 GI; 1 g Prot.; 18 g
Carb.; 0 g SFA; 0 g MUFA; 0 g PUFA; 0 g
Omega-3; 13 mg Calc.; 3 mg Sod.; 117 mg
Pot.; 0 mg Iron; 0 mg Phytoestrogen; 3 g Fiber

Preheat the oven to 350°F.

Peel, halve, and core the pears. Place them cut side down in a rectangular baking dish with just enough water to cover the bottom of the dish.

Combine the sugar with the spices and sprinkle half of this mixture over the pears. Bake the pears for 5 minutes in the preheated oven. Turn the pear halves over, sprinkle with the remaining spice mixture, and continue to bake for another 5 minutes. The pears are done when they are easily pierced by a fork but still hold their shape. Large pears may take a little longer to cook. Remove from the oven, place in individual dessert dishes, and set aside.

To make the sauce, combine the egg yolk and sugar in a very small saucepan and mix vigorously for at least 5 minutes with a wooden spoon. Slowly add the Marsala and mix well. Heat over low heat, stirring constantly, for about 1 minute, or until the mixture thickens. Do not let it come to a boil. Pour the sauce over the pear halves and serve warm or at room temperature.

Watermelon Granita

When you're too hot to handle, try relaxing and enjoy this cooling, refreshing frozen dessert. Also called Italian ices, granitas can also be made with other fruits, such as lemon, pink grapefruit, and strawberries.

Yield: 4 servings

Simple Syrup:
1 cup sugar

Granita:
4 cups seedless watermelon chunks
1 cup simple syrup (above)
Juice of 1 lemon

To make the simple syrup, bring 1 cup of water to a boil in a saucepan. Add the sugar and cook until dissolved. Once the sugar is dissolved completely, remove the saucepan from the heat and set aside to cool fully.

To make the granita, combine the watermelon, simple syrup, and lemon juice in a food processor. Puree until smooth. Pour into a 9 by 13-inch plastic or glass container and freeze for 1 hour. Rake the mixture with a fork and freeze for another hour. Check it a few times to make sure it does not freeze completely. Rake and freeze for 1 more hour. Rake and serve in cups. (The texture should be granular.)

—*Rachel Giblin*

Per serving: 147 Cal.; 64 GI; 1 g Prot.; 37 g Carb.; 0 g SFA; 0 g MUFA; 0 g PUFA; 0 g Omega-3; 16 mg Calc.; 3 mg Sod.; 191 mg Pot.; 4 mg Iron; 0 mg Phytoestrogen; 1 g Fiber

Fruit Flambé over Sorbet

This is a great dessert for a party because it's fast and the guests will love the show. It's a nice light dessert that everyone will love, and it's somewhat guiltless.

Yield: 4 servings

2 bananas, cut into ½-inch slices

½ pint strawberries, hulled and quartered

¼ cup agave syrup

⅓ cup Grand Marnier or Malibu coconut rum

6 scoops raspberry sorbet, three-flavored swirl, or low-fat vanilla ice cream

Put the bananas, strawberries, and agave syrup in a saucepan over medium-low heat and cook for about 1 minute. Remove the pan from the heat and pour in the Grand Marnier. Lower the heat to low and carefully place the saucepan back on the heat (the alcohol will ignite and flame up for a second; stand back so you don't burn your hair or clothing) and cook until the fruit is tender but not mushy. Scoop the sorbet into six individual serving bowls and pour the fruit mixture over the top. Serve immediately.

—Will Greenwood

Per serving: 291 Cal.; 67 GI; 1 g Prot.; 64 g Carb.; 0 g SFA; 0 g MUFA; 0.1 g PUFA; 0 g Omega-3; 27 mg Calc.; 12 mg Sod.; 332 mg Pot.; 1 mg Iron; 0 mg Phytoestrogen; 3 g Fiber

Baked Alaska

This is a festival traditional dessert that can be served with low-fat ice cream. It is fun to present and can be made ahead of time. What more could you ask?

Yield: 6 servings

Swiss Meringue:
5 egg whites
½ cup agave syrup

Cake:
1 (½-gallon) container of your favorite sorbet or low-fat ice cream
Angel food cake, store-bought or made ahead of time (a cake mix works well)

Variations:

This recipe can also be formed into individual cakes for each person.

To make the meringue, take the eggs out of the refrigerator for 45 minutes to come to room temperature. Separate the yolks from the whites, making sure there is no yolk at all in the whites (any fat or oil will prevent the meringue from forming).

Put the egg whites and agave syrup in a mixing bowl. Place a medium-size pot of hot water on the stove over medium heat and place the mixing bowl over the pot. Whip constantly until the egg whites are warm to the touch, 110° to 120°F. You may need to adjust the heat; if it is too high, you may cook the whites.

To make the cake, take the sorbet out of the freezer to soften it slightly. When the whites and syrup are warmed through, place in the bowl of an electric mixer and whip on high speed until you have a very thick meringue. Set aside.

Cut the cake into the shape of the serving plate you will use, to form a base about ¼ inch thick or slightly thicker. (This can have seams and be pieced together, as nobody will see it.) Spread a layer of the sorbet about 5 inches thick on top of this base. With the remaining cake, cut pieces to form a layer about ¼ inch thick and place on top of the sorbet.

Fill a piping bag with the meringue and, using a small knife, ice the cake with the meringue, allowing peaks and spikes to form, because this will make it beautiful when it is heated and browned. You can pipe decorations around the base and on the cake if you like. Have fun making it with the kids, because there are no mistakes with baked Alaska.

After the cake is iced, place it in the freezer for at least 4 to 5 hours before serving. You can make this up to 4 days ahead of time. The cake needs to be very solid in order to brown it. Restaurants use torches, but a broiler or even the oven will work well. If a torch is used, which is the easiest way, take the cake out 15 to 20 minutes before serving to temper the sorbet.

Light the torch and go over the entire cake, browning everything that has a peak. If the broiler is used, temper it the same way, but put the cake under the broiler, watching carefully and rotating it; don't let any part burn (This is hardest way to brown it). The second easiest way is in the oven. Preheat the oven to 450°F for 20 minutes, and then take the cake directly from the freezer, place it in the oven, bake until it is browned all over. If this method is used, you should not make the peaks so high. (You can use a star-shaped tip for decorating so that there aren't any large peaks to burn.) When all the peaks are browned, cut the cake into serving portions and enjoy this classic updated version of hot and cold bliss.

—Will Greenwood

Per serving: 687 Cal.; 69 GI; 10 g Prot.; 167 g Carb.; 0 g SFA; 0 g MUFA; 0.1 g PUFA; 0 g Omega-3; 38 mg Calc.; 817 mg Sod.; 348 mg Pot.; 2 mg Iron; 0 mg Phytoestrogen; 1.5 g Fiber

Frozen Berry Yogurt

Anneka Manning's frozen yogurt from the Low GI Family Cookbook *is easy to prepare and perfect for summery desserts. You can refreeze it in single-serving containers in the final step rather than in one large container, if you prefer, and have it on hand as an after-school or after-work snack.*

Yield: 6 servings

9 ounces fresh or frozen mixed berries

3 (7-ounce) tubs low-fat vanilla yogurt

2 egg whites

2 tablespoons pure floral honey

Place the berries and yogurt in a food processor and blend until smooth. Transfer to a medium-size bowl and set aside.

Whisk the egg whites in a clean, dry bowl until stiff peaks form. Add the honey, a tablespoon at a time, whisking well after each addition until thick and glossy. Fold into the yogurt mixture until just combined.

Pour the mixture into an airtight container and place in the freezer for 4 hours, or until frozen. Use a metal spoon to break the frozen yogurt into chunks. Blend again in a food processor until smooth. Return to the airtight container and refreeze for 3 hours, or until frozen. Serve in scoops.

—University of Sydney Glycemic Index and GI Database

Per serving: 126 Cal.; 43 GI; 6 g Prot.; 23 g Carb.; 1 g SFA; 0.3 g MUFA; 0 g PUFA; 0 g Omega-3; 178 mg Calc.; 85 mg Sod.; 302 mg Pot.; 0.5 mg Iron; 0 mg Phytoestrogen; 1 g Fiber

Mock Apple Pie

This recipe will leave your guests wanting more of the best apple pie ever. You may even enjoy not telling them that there aren't any apples in the recipe.

Yield: 6 servings (1 pie)

3 cups zucchini, peeled, seeded, and sliced thinly

3 tablespoons lemon juice

1 teaspoon ground cinnamon

½ cup granulated sugar

½ cup brown sugar

3 tablespoons all-purpose flour

Pastry for one 9-inch double-crusted pie

1 tablespoon butter, cut into small pieces (optional)

Preheat the oven to 350°F.

Place the zucchini slices in a mixing bowl and sprinkle with the lemon juice. Combine the cinnamon, sugars, and flour in a small bowl and stir into the zucchini mixture.

Place one piecrust in the bottom of a 9-inch pie pan. Spread the zucchini mixture in the pan and dot with the butter, if using. Place the other piecrust on top and seal and flute. Bake for 45 minutes, or until the zucchini is tender and the crust is lightly browned.

—*Cynthia Niles*

Per serving: 223 Cal.; 63 GI; 2 g Prot.; 43 g Carb.; 1.5 g SFA; 3 g MUFA; 1 g PUFA; 0.3 g Omega-3; 31 mg Calc.; 44 mg Sod.; 193 mg Pot.; 1 mg Iron; 0 mg Phytoestrogen; 1 g Fiber

Get Off the Sugar Roller Coaster

Avoid sugar blasts such as doughnuts, sweetened soda, and candy. They send your blood sugar up and down quickly and bring your mood with it. Reach for a piece of fruit or a carrot stick. Just sucking on a hard candy may allow the urge to splurge to pass.

Chocolate Mousse Pie

This rich-tasting, luxurious wheat-free (though not gluten-free) chocolate mousse pie is great for any occasion. For an excellent variation, make it with a combination of chocolate and peanut butter chips.

Yield: 8 servings (1 pie)

Piecrust:

1 cup spelt flour

¼ cup unsweetened cocoa powder

¼ cup Sucanat

1 teaspoon baking powder

1 teaspoon baking soda

½ cup soy milk

½ cup pure maple syrup

¼ cup safflower oil

½ teaspoon vanilla extract

¼ teaspoon almond extract

2 tablespoons chocolate chips

Mousse:

2¼ cups chocolate chips

1 cup plus 2 tablespoons vanilla soy milk

½ teaspoon unsweetened cocoa powder

½ teaspoon kudzu

1¼ (20-ounce) blocks silken tofu

¼ cup pure maple syrup

2 teaspoons vanilla extract

1 teaspoon almond extract

To prepare the piecrust, preheat the oven to 325°F. Mix the flour, cocoa powder, Sucanat, baking powder, and baking soda together in a large mixing bowl. In another bowl, combine the soy milk, maple syrup, oil, ½ cup of water, and the vanilla and almond extracts. Add the wet ingredients to the flour mixture and stir well to combine. Pour the mixture into a 9-inch pie pan and bake for 35 minutes. Let cool in the refrigerator for about 1 hour.

Crumble the baked dough and press the crust crumbs into a 9-inch pie dish and sprinkle with the chocolate chips.

To prepare the mousse filling, place the chocolate chips, 1 cup of the soy milk, and the cocoa powder in a bowl. Dissolve the kudzu in the remaining 2 tablespoons of soy milk and add to the mixture. Place the mixture in a double boiler and heat over simmering water over medium heat until melted, stirring occasionally. Transfer to a mixing bowl and let cool slightly.

Place the tofu in a food processor and blend until smooth. Add the maple syrup, vanilla, and almond extracts and blend again. Fold into the chocolate mixture until well blended. Pour the chocolate mixture into the piecrust and chill for up to 2 hours or overnight before serving.

—*Benay Vynerib*

Per serving (mousse): 354 Cal.; 34 GI; 8 g Prot.; 40 g Carb.; 9 g SFA; 5 g MUFA; 2 g PUFA; 0.1 g Omega-3; 94 mg Calc.; 55 mg Sod.; 469 mg Pot.; 5 mg Iron; 24 mg Phytoestrogen; 4 g Fiber

Per serving (crust): 223 Cal.; 59 GI; 5 g Prot.; 34 g Carb.; 1 g SFA; 1.5 g MUFA; 5.5 g PUFA; 0 g Omega-3; 97 mg Calc.; 275 mg Sod.; 203 mg Pot.; 2 mg Iron; 2 mg Phytoestrogen; 3 g Fiber

Best Carrot Cake Ever

This is a delicious cake. Enjoy it as a special treat! Carrots are a great source of fiber and vitamin C.

Yield: 12 servings

Cake:
2 cups whole wheat flour
1¾ cups sugar
2 teaspoons baking soda
1 teaspoon baking powder
1 teaspoon salt
2 teaspoons ground cinnamon
½ cup oil
½ cup applesauce
3 egg whites
1 teaspoon vanilla extract
1 (8-ounce) can crushed pineapple, drained
2 cups shredded carrots
1 cup flaked coconut
1 cup chopped walnuts

Cream Cheese Frosting:
1 (8-ounce) package light cream cheese
¼ cup butter (½ stick), at room temperature
2 cups confectioners' sugar
1½ teaspoons vanilla extract
Splash of milk, if needed

Preheat the oven to 350°F. Grease and flour a 13 by 9 by 2-inch baking pan.

To make the cake, combine the flour, sugar, baking soda, baking powder, salt, and cinnamon in a large mixing bowl and mix well. Make a well in the center of the mixture.

In another bowl, combine the oil, applesauce, egg whites, vanilla, pineapple, and carrots and mix well. Pour this mixture into the well in the center of the dry ingredients and mix until well combined.

Once the batter is mixed, fold in the coconut and walnuts and spoon into the prepared baking pan. Bake for 45 minutes, or until the cake springs back when pressed lightly in the center with your fingertip.

To make the cream cheese frosting, while the cake is baking, combine the cheese, butter, sugar, and vanilla in a mixing bowl and mix well, adding a little milk if needed to make a spreadable consistency (you can use a hand mixer if you have one).

Best Carrot Cake Ever (continued)

When the cake is done, put the pan on a wire rack until the cake cools to room temperature. When cool, carefully turn the cake out onto a serving plate, spread the frosting over the top, and serve.

—Kristin Denice

Per serving (cake): 393 Cal.; 55 GI; 6 g Prot.; 52 g Carb.; 5 g SFA; 7 g MUFA; 7 g PUFA; 2 g Omega-3; 55 mg Calc.; 373 mg Sod.; 267 mg Pot.; 1.5 mg Iron; 0 mg Phytoestrogen; 5 g Fiber

Per serving (frosting): 151 Cal.; 59 GI; 1.5 g Prot.; 21 g Carb.; 4 g SFA; 1 g MUFA; 0 g PUFA; 0 g Omega-3; 29 mg Calc.; 116 mg Sod.; 49 mg Pot.; 0 mg Iron; 0 mg Phytoestrogen; 0 g Fiber

Dewberry's Triple Chocolate Brownies

These are delicious but rich treats, so enjoy one and alternate with other desserts, such as berries. Flaxseeds are a great source of dietary fiber, calcium, iron, and omega-3 fatty acids.

Yield: 12 brownies

4 ounces unsweetened baking chocolate

¼ pound butter (1 stick)

½ cup all-purpose flour

½ cup whole wheat flour

¼ cup milled flaxseeds

¼ teaspoon sea salt

1 cup chopped walnuts or pecans

1 cup chopped bittersweet or semisweet chocolate chips

2 cups granulated or raw sugar

2 tablespoons Ghirardelli sweet ground chocolate and cocoa, or unsweetened cocoa powder

4 eggs

1 teaspoon vanilla extract

Preheat the oven to 325°F. Line a 9 by 13 by 2-inch baking pan with parchment or waxed paper.

In a heavy saucepan, melt the baking chocolate and butter. Set aside to cool for at least 10 minutes.

Put the flours, flaxseeds, and salt in a mixing bowl and mix well. Put the nuts and chocolate chips in another bowl and add a tablespoon of the flour mixture. Toss well to coat. Put the sugar and cocoa powder in a large mixing bowl and add the eggs, one at a time, whisking to mix, but do not overmix. Stir in the vanilla. When the chocolate and butter mixture has cooled, add it to the egg mixture and mix well. Add the flour mixture and mix well, and then fold in the chocolate chips and nuts.

Spread the batter in the prepared pan and bake for 30 to 35 minutes, or until a toothpick comes out mostly clean. If you cook it until the center is completely cooked, it will be overdone and dry.

Let cool in the pan for an hour. Run a knife around the edge and turn out onto a rack. Transfer to a cutting board, flipping it to the other side, and cut into twelve pieces. The top is going to crack, so be ready for it. That's the charm of these brownies. They will have a crunchy top and chewy center.

—Jeffrey Parker

Per serving: 458 Cal.; 59 GI; 7 g Prot.; 56 g Carb.; 12 g SFA; 7 g MUFA; 6 g PUFA; 1.5 g Omega-3; 44 mg Calc.; 133 mg Sod.; 253 mg Pot.; 3 mg Iron; 0 mg Phytoestrogen; 4.5 g Fiber

Chocolate Zucchini Bread

This is a delicious way to use the abundance of zucchini available in the warm weather. The bread freezes well.

Yield: 3 loaves, serving 24 (8 servings per loaf)

3 cups whole wheat flour

3 cups sugar

½ cup unsweetened cocoa powder

1½ teaspoons baking powder

1½ teaspoons baking soda

1 teaspoon salt

¼ teaspoon ground cinnamon

4 eggs

1½ cups vegetable oil

2 teaspoons butter, melted

1½ teaspoons vanilla extract

1½ teaspoons almond extract

3 cups grated zucchini

1 cup chopped nuts

Preheat the oven to 350°F. Grease and flour three 8 by 4 by 2½-inch loaf pans.

Combine the flour, sugar, cocoa, baking powder, baking soda, salt, and cinnamon in a large mixing bowl and mix well. In a separate bowl, combine the eggs, oil, butter, and extracts and mix well. Stir the egg mixture into the dry ingredients until moistened, and then fold in the zucchini and nuts. Pour the mixture into the prepared loaf pans and bake for 70 minutes, or until a toothpick inserted in the center comes out clean.

Remove from the oven and let cool for 10 minutes before removing the loaves from the pans.

—*Cynthia Niles*

Per serving: 323 Cal.; 57 GI; 4 g Prot.; 38 g Carb.; 3 g SFA; 10 g MUFA; 5 g PUFA; 1.5 g Omega-3; 34 mg Calc.; 227 mg Sod.; 144 mg Pot.; 1 mg Iron; 0 mg Phytoestrogen; 3 g Fiber

Mandelbrodt

There is no doubt in my mind that this is my favorite cookie. It's not too sweet, it lasts forever in a canister, and it's perfect for any occasion. To change the taste, add 1 cup of raisins, ¾ cup of chocolate chips, or ½ cup of chopped walnuts to the dough.

Yield: About 60 cookies (2 cookies per serving)

Cooking spray
3 eggs
Pinch of salt
I cup plus 2 tablespoons sugar
¾ cup oil
I teaspoon vanilla extract
I teaspoon almond extract
3½ cups whole wheat flour
3 teaspoons baking powder
2 tablespoons ground cinnamon

Preheat the oven to 350°F. Spray a cookie sheet with cooking spray.

In a small mixing bowl, beat the eggs and add the salt, 1 cup of the sugar, and the oil and extracts. Mix well. Combine the flour and baking powder in a large mixing bowl and mix well, and then add the egg mixture to the flour mixture and mix until completely combined.

Divide the batter into four or five equal portions and roll into "logs" and flatten slightly. Combine the remaining 2 tablespoons of sugar and the cinnamon and spread on a sheet of waxed paper. Roll the logs in the mixture to lightly coat, and then lay them on the prepared cookie sheet about 1 inch apart. Place in the oven and bake for 30 minutes.

Remove from the oven and cut each log into ½-inch slices. Turn the cookies onto their side and leave on the cookie sheet.

Turn off the oven and return the cookies to oven until the oven is cool and the cookies are crisp.

—Bubbie's Kitchen

Per serving: 133 Cal.; 53 GI; 2 g Prot.; 18 g Carb.; 0.5 g SFA; 4 g MUFA; 2 g PUFA; 0.5 g Omega-3; 39 mg Calc.; 95 mg Sod.; 66 mg Pot.; 1 mg Iron; 0 mg Phytoestrogen; 2 g Fiber

Oatmeal Chocolate Chip Cookies

These healthy, vegan, wheat-free (though not gluten-free) cookies are made at the juice bar in the Candle Café and Candle 79 in New York City, and they fly out of the restaurant as soon as they are made.

Yield: 18 cookies (2 cookies per serving)

1 cup rolled oats

1 cup spelt flour

¼ cup brown rice flour

¼ teaspoon baking soda

¼ teaspoon fine sea salt

¾ cup safflower oil

1 cup pure maple syrup

¼ teaspoon vanilla extract

¼ teaspoon almond extract (optional)

1 tablespoon egg replacer

1 cup chocolate chips

Preheat the oven to 350°F.

Combine the oats, flours, baking soda, and salt in a large mixing bowl. Add the oil, ¼ cup of water, maple syrup, vanilla and almond extracts, and the egg replacer and stir well to combine.

Fold the chocolate chips into the batter.

Spoon tablespoons of batter 3 inches apart onto a large baking sheet. Flatten the batter with the back of a wet spoon. Bake for 10 to 15 minutes, until lightly browned. Remove the cookies from the baking sheet and let cool on wire racks.

—*Benay Vynerib*

Per serving: 288 Cal.; 46 GI; 3 g Prot.; 35 g Carb.; 3 g SFA; 3 g MUFA; 8 g PUFA; 0 g Omega-3; 29 mg Calc.; 68 mg Sod.; 192 mg Pot.; 2 mg Iron; 0 mg Phytoestrogen; 3 g Fiber

Mango Lassi

This cooling yogurt drink is a great source of dietary fiber and vitamins B$_6$, A, and C; and yogurt is a great source of calcium. It's both healthy and very refreshing.

Yield: 4 to 6 servings

2 medium-size very ripe mangoes, peeled and sliced

2 cups low-fat, plain yogurt

2 tablespoons pure maple syrup or honey

6 ice cubes

8 teaspoons rose water

Place the mango slices, yogurt, maple syrup, ice cubes, and rose water in the bowl of a food processor. Process at high speed until well blended. Serve immediately.

—Dr. Mache's Kitchen

Per serving: 571 Cal.; 47 GI; 5 g Prot.; 26 g Carb.; 1 g SFA; 0.5 g MUFA; 0 g PUFA; 0 g Omega-3; 193 mg Calc.; 71 mg Sod.; 375 mg Pot.; 0.2 mg Iron; 0 mg Phytoestrogen; 1.5 g Fiber

Golden Milk

Golden milk is a delicious hot drink that the yogis believe is good for your joints and spine. They also believe it is a good nightcap and calming for women.

Yield: I serving

⅛ teaspoon turmeric

I cup 1% milk

2 teaspoons raw almond oil (be sure to use culinary, not cosmetic, oil)

½ teaspoon honey

Put the turmeric and ¼ cup of water in a small saucepan and boil for about 8 minutes, until it forms a thick paste. If too much water boils away, add a little more. Meanwhile, in another saucepan, bring the milk and almond oil just to a boil. As soon as it boils, remove it from the heat. Combine the two mixtures in a large mug and stir in the honey to taste. This is delicious hot or cold.

You can also blend in a food processor until frothy, and add a sprinkle of cinnamon.

—Hari Kaur Khalsa

Per serving: 178 Cal.; 43 GI; 4 g Prot.; 7 g Carb.; 2 g SFA; 10 g MUFA; 2 g PUFA; 0 g Omega-3; 146 mg Calc.; 55 mg Sod.; 147 mg Pot.; 0.1 mg Iron; 0 mg Phytoestrogen; 0 g Fiber

METRIC CONVERSION CHART

- The recipes in this book have not been tested with metric measurements, so some variations might occur.
- Remember that the weight of dry ingredients varies according to the volume or density factor: 1 cup of flour weighs far less than 1 cup of sugar, and 1 tablespoon doesn't necessarily hold 3 teaspoons.

General Formulas for Metric Conversion

Ounces to grams	$\Rightarrow$ ounces × 28.35 = grams
Grams to ounces	$\Rightarrow$ grams × 0.035 = ounces
Pounds to grams	$\Rightarrow$ pounds × 453.5 = grams
Pounds to kilograms	$\Rightarrow$ pounds × 0.45 = kilograms
Cups to liters	$\Rightarrow$ cups × 0.24 = liters
Fahrenheit to Celsius	$\Rightarrow$ (°F – 32) × 5 ÷ 9 = °C
Celsius to Fahrenheit	$\Rightarrow$ (°C × 9) ÷ 5 + 32 = °F

Linear Measurements

½ inch = 1½ cm
1 inch = 2½ cm
6 inches = 15 cm
8 inches = 20 cm
10 inches = 25 cm
12 inches = 30 cm
20 inches = 50 cm

Volume (Dry) Measurements

¼ teaspoon = 1 milliliter
½ teaspoon = 2 milliliters
¾ teaspoon = 4 milliliters
1 teaspoon = 5 milliliters
1 tablespoon = 15 milliliters
¼ cup = 59 milliliters
⅓ cup = 79 milliliters
½ cup = 118 milliliters
⅔ cup = 158 milliliters
¾ cup = 177 milliliters
1 cup = 225 milliliters
4 cups or 1 quart = 1 liter
½ gallon = 2 liters
1 gallon = 4 liters

Volume (Liquid) Measurements

1 teaspoon = ⅙ fluid ounce = 5 milliliters
1 tablespoon = ½ fluid ounce = 15 milliliters
2 tablespoons = 1 fluid ounce = 30 milliliters
¼ cup = 2 fluid ounces = 60 milliliters
⅓ cup = 2⅔ fluid ounces = 79 milliliters
½ cup = 4 fluid ounces = 118 milliliters
1 cup or ½ pint = 8 fluid ounces = 250 milliliters
2 cups or 1 pint = 16 fluid ounces = 500 milliliters
4 cups or 1 quart = 32 fluid ounces = 1,000 milliliters
1 gallon = 4 liters

Oven Temperature Equivalents, Fahrenheit (F) and Celsius (C)

100°F = 38°C
200°F = 95°C
250°F = 120°C
300°F = 150°C
350°F = 180°C
400°F = 205°C
450°F = 230°C

Weight (Mass) Measurements

1 ounce = 30 grams
2 ounces = 55 grams
3 ounces = 85 grams
4 ounces = ¼ pound = 125 grams
8 ounces = ½ pound = 240 grams
12 ounces = ¾ pound = 375 grams
16 ounces = 1 pound = 454 grams

APPENDIX

VITAMINS AND MINERALS FOR A HEALTHY DIET*

VITAMIN / MINERAL	POSSIBLE BENEFITS	DIETARY SOURCES	CONCERNS
Vitamin A (beta-carotene) RDA Women: 4,000 IU Men: 5,000 IU	Essential for normal growth and for eye and skin health. Helps you see at night.	Carrots, dark green leafy vegetables, cantaloupe, and peaches, as well as liver, eggs, milk, and butter.	Beta-carotene is converted in the body to vitamin A. Generally safe up to 10,000 IU daily. May be toxic above 50,000 IU. Doses above 20,000 IU daily during pregnancy may cause birth defects, but not everyone agrees this is so. High dosages may increase the risk of lung cancer in smokers.
Vitamin B$_3$ (Niacin) RDA Women: 14 mg Pregnant women: 18 mg Men: 16 mg	Helps process fat, produce blood sugar, and get rid of waste materials from tissue. Niacin also helps reduce blood cholesterol levels, which reduces the risk of heart disease.	Can be found in meats, but can also be made in the body from the proteins found in eggs and milk. Often added to the flour in breads and pasta.	Safe up to 35 mg daily. Niacin supplements can cause itching, tingling, rashes, and occasionally a feeling of intense heat. Very high dosages of niacin can cause liver damage.

Continues . . .

*Adapted from M. M. Seibel and H. K. Khalsa, *A Woman's Book of Yoga* (New York: Penguin Putnam, 2002).

VITAMIN / MINERAL	POSSIBLE BENEFITS	DIETARY SOURCES	CONCERNS
Vitamin B₆ (pyridoxine) RDA Adults to age 50: 1.3 mg Pregnant women: 2.0 mg Women over 50: 1.5 mg Men over 50: 1.7 mg	Helps the body process fats, proteins, and carbohydrates, as well as build red blood cells and the immune system. May help prevent heart disease. Women in the United States consume less than the RDA.	Meats, liver, enriched grains, eggs, bananas, and peanut butter.	Dosages above 200 mg daily for several months could lead to numbness in the hands and feet and difficulty walking.
Vitamin B₁₂ (Cyanocobalamin) RDA Adults: 2.4 mcg Pregnant women: 2.6 mcg	Essential for normal cell development, especially blood cells, and protein synthesis. Helps the body use fats and carbohydrates and helps the nervous system work properly.	Meat, fish, eggs, chicken, and dairy products.	Generally without risk in dosages up to 100 mcg. Individuals with abnormal intestinal absorption and strict vegetarians may become B₁₂ deficient during pregnancy, especially if they breast-feed.
Vitamin C RDA Adults: 60 mg	Antioxidant, protects cells from natural deterioration that results from aging. Also necessary to produce collagen, which makes up connective tissue.	Fresh fruits (especially citrus) and vegetables, green vegetables, tomatoes, and potatoes.	Dosages up to 1,000 mg probably without risk. Higher dosages may cause diarrhea. Drying, salting, or cooking (especially in copper pots), mincing of fresh vegetables, or mashing potatoes reduces the amount of vitamin C in foods. Pregnant women, smokers, and excessive alcohol consumers benefit from extra vitamin C.
Vitamin D RDA Adults to age 50: 200 IU Adults 51–70: 400 IU Adults over 70: 600–800 IU	Important regulator of the repair and formation of bone. Also controls calcium and phosphorous absorption from food.	Milk is the most important source. Exposure to at least 15 minutes of sunlight without a sunscreen also allows your body to form vitamin D. Older men and women and people living in areas where the days are short probably need a daily supplement of vitamin D.	Dosages up to 2,000 IU are safe. More than 5,000 IU daily can lead to kidney damage unless you are deficient. People in nursing homes or who do not get outside and women in menopause and with osteoporosis should consider supplementing with vitamin D.

VITAMIN / MINERAL	POSSIBLE BENEFITS	DIETARY SOURCES	CONCERNS
Vitamin E RDA Adults: 30 IU	Antioxidant that protects cells from natural deterioration. Helps reduce risk of heart disease and blood clots. Involved in making red blood cells.	Richest sources include salad dressing, cooking oils, and margarine, which together provide 30 percent of vitamin E in the American diet. Other sources include almonds, filberts, Brazil nuts, wheat-germ oil, sunflower seeds, corn, asparagus, avocados, organ meats, butter, and eggs.	Studies have shown safety at doses of 800 IU daily. Dosages of at least 100 IU daily appear to have a major potential to reduce the risk of heart attack.
Folic Acid RDA Adults: 400 mcg Pregnant women: up to 800 mcg	A member of the B-complex family, helps reduce the risk of heart disease. Helps reduce women's risk of having a baby with a neurological birth defect. Needed for normal red blood cell development.	Raw leafy green vegetables, peas and beans, citrus fruits, and fortified cereals.	The average American consumes only 200 mcg of folic acid daily, and cooking removes more than half of the folic acid in food. Pregnant women with a history of miscarriage or of preeclampsia (a type of high blood pressure in pregnancy) or who take antiseizure medications may benefit from 800 mcg daily. More than 1,000 mcg daily may cause zinc loss or mask B_{12} deficiency.
Calcium RDA Children/Young adults: 1–10 yrs: 800–1,200 mg 11–24 yrs: 1,200–1,500 mg Adult women: Pregnant/lactating: 1,200–1,500 mg 25–49 yrs: 1,000 mg 50–64 yrs. taking estrogen: 1,000 mg 50–64 yrs. not on estrogen: 1,500 mg	Promotes healthy bones, prevents osteoporosis, and helps keep teeth strong. Also essential for muscle contraction and relaxation.	Milk, cheese, yogurt, leafy greens, broccoli, tofu, sardines (especially with bones), and salmon. If you don't eat much of these foods or are lactose intolerant, take a supplement.	Safe up to 2,500 mg daily. May reduce absorption of zinc and iron. Higher dosages can cause kidney stones, so be sure to drink 8 glasses of water daily. The mineral calcium is combined with one of several salts when taken as a supplement. These include calcium carbonate, calcium citrate, and calcium phosphate. **Continues . . .**

VITAMIN / MINERAL	POSSIBLE BENEFITS	DIETARY SOURCES	CONCERNS
Calcium (continued) RDA Adult women: 65+ yrs.: 1,500 mg Adult men 25–64 yrs.: 1,000 mg 65+ yrs.: 1,500 mg			Calcium carbonate is the least expensive but is less well absorbed. Calcium citrate and phosphate are absorbed more readily.
Chromium RDA Adults: 50–200 mcg	Helps convert blood sugar into energy. Helps insulin work effectively, so may help prevent diabetes.	Healthy amounts found in peanuts and beer, cheese, broccoli, wheat germ, and liver.	Not recommended above 200 mcg daily.
Iron RDA Women: 15 mg Men: 10 mg Pregnant women: 30 mg	Necessary for making red blood cells and hemoglobin.	Abundant in meats, eggs, lentils, nuts, leafy green vegetables, Cheddar cheese, and mussels.	Believed safe up to 75 mg daily. Needs to be reduced drastically in menopause. Absorption of iron may interfere with absorption of zinc, copper, and calcium. When taking supplemental iron, add 15 mg of zinc and 2 mg of copper. Insufficient iron is a common cause of anemia, especially in children and women of reproductive age due to poor dietary intake.
Zinc RDA Women: 12 mg Men: 15 mg	Helps red blood cells carry carbon dioxide to the lungs for disposal. Helps wound healing and keeping the senses alert. May help prevent colds and reduce risk of premature delivery toward the end of pregnancy.	Abundant in red meats, bread and other grain products, eggs, milk, sunflower seeds, soybeans, chicken, and seafood (especially oysters).	Safe up to 30 mg daily. 2,000 mg daily can lead to vomiting.

RECIPE CONTRIBUTORS

Aldo, Chef
Riverside Country Club
2500 Springhill Road
Bozeman, MT 59718
Tel.: 406-587-5105

Antonio Laudisio
Laudisio Italian Restaurant
1710 29th Street
Boulder, CO 80301

Aviva Goldfarb
The Six O'clock Scramble
Chevy Chase, MD
www.thescramble.com

Ben Schwendener
Gravity Arts Studio
Jamaica Plain, MA
www.BenSchwendener.com

Benay Vynerib, COO
Candle Café and Candle 79
1307 Third Avenue
New York, NY 10021-3301
Tel.: 212-472-0970 /
212-537-7179
E-mail:
Benay@candlecafe.com
www.candlecafe.com

Bill Hart, Chef
Black Dog Café
Martha's Vineyard, MA

Brad Parsons, Chef
Fairmont Chicago,
Millennium Park
200 North Columbus Drive
Chicago, IL 60601

Brad Stevens, Executive Chef
Community Servings
Jamaica Plain, MA
Tel.: 617-522-7777
www.servings.org

**Bubbie's Kitchen
(Elaine Seibel)**
Houston, TX

Carrie Nahabedian
NAHA Restaurant, Chicago
500 North Clark Street
Chicago, IL 60654
Tel.: 312-321-6242

Catherine D'Amato
Greater Boston Food Bank
70 South Bay Avenue
Boston, MA 02118

Cathy Whims, Chef
Nostrana
1401 SE Morrison
Portland, OR 97214
E-mail: nostrana@gmail.com

Cynthia Niles
Red Hot Mamas
Charlestown, RI

Donnie Ferneau Jr., CEC
Ferneau Restaurant
2601 Kavanaugh Blvd.
Little Rock, AR 72205
Tel.: 501-603-9208
www.ferneaurestaurant.com

Dr. Mache's Kitchen
(Mache Seibel)
233 Needham Street, Suite 300
Newton, MA 02464

Gordon Hamersley
Hamersley's Bistro
553 Tremont Street
Boston, MA 02118
E-mail: Ghamersley3@aol.com

Hari Kaur Khalsa
New York, NY
www.reachhari.com

**Heather Tsatsarones,
MS, RD, LDN**
Community Servings
Jamaica Plain, MA
Tel.: 617-522-7777
www.servings.org

Jason Franey, Chef
Canlis Restaurant
2576 Aurora Avenue North
Seattle, WA 98109
Tel: 206-283-3313
www.canlis.com

Jeffrey S. Merry, Chef
Agar Supply
225 John Hancock Road
Taunton, MA 02780-7318
Tel.: 617-880-5164
E-mail: jmerry@agarsupply.com

Jeffrey Parker
Former contestant on
Hell's Kitchen
The Flying Biscuit Café
Atlanta, GA
www.flyingbiscuit.com

Joanne Choi
Week of Menus
www.weekofmenus.com

John Liberatore
Liberatore's Restaurant
9515 Deereco Road
Timonium, MD 21093
Tel: 410-561-3300
Fax: 410-561-2404

Jonathan Cartwright, Chef
The White Barn Inn
37 Beach Avenue
Kennebunk Beach, ME 04043
E-mail: jonathan.cartwright@
ushotelsgroup.com

Karen's Cucina
(Karen Giblin)
Tel.: 908-704-2184
E-mail: kgiblin@redhot
mamas.org

Kristin Denice
The Schoolhouse B&B
119 Boon Street
Narragansett, RI 02882

Kristin Wilson
Hamersley's Bistro
553 Tremont Street
Boston, MA 02118

Luis Bollo, Chef
Meigas Restaurant
10 Wall Street
Norwalk, CT 06850
Tel.: 203-866-8800
Contact: Mario Aguilar
E-mail: m2a2forever@
yahoo.com

**Michael Fiorello,
Chef de Cuisine**
Mercat a la Planxa
638 South Michigan Avenue
Chicago, IL 60605
www.mercatchicago.com

Michelle Bernstein
Michy's
6927 Biscayne Blvd.
Miami, FL 33138
Tel.: 305-759-2001

Neal Fraser, Chef
Grace Restaurant
7360 Beverly Blvd.
Los Angeles, CA 90036-2501
E-mail: neal@
gracerestaurant.com

Rachel Giblin
Red Hot Mamas
Bozeman, MT 59715
E-mail: rjgiblin@redhot
mamas.org

**Tony Murillo,
Kitchen Manager**
Community Servings
Jamaica Plain, MA
Tel.: 617-522-7777
www.servings.org

Tres Hundertmark, Chef
The Lobster Trap
35 Patton Avenue
Asheville, NC 28801
Tel.: 828-350-0505
E-mail: tres@thelobstertrap.biz

**University of Sydney Glycemic
Index and GI Database**
Sydney, Australia
www.glycemicindex.com

**Will Greenwood,
Chef Consultant**
E-mail: Chefgreenwood
@aol.com
www.myspace.com/chefwill
greenwood.com

NOTES

Introduction

1. M. M. Seibel, *The Soy Solution for Menopause: The Estrogen Alternative* (New York: Simon & Schuster, 2003).

Chapter 1: A Little About Perimenopause and Menopause

1. NAMS, *Menopause Practice: A Clinician's Guide*, 4th ed., 2010, 1.2.

2. Ibid., 4.9.

3. M. M. Seibel, *The Soy Solution for Menopause: The Estrogen Alternative* (New York: Simon & Schuster, 2003).

4. M. M. Seibel and H. K. Khalsa, *A Woman's Book of Yoga* (New York: Penguin Putnam, 2002).

Chapter 2: What Does "Healthy Weight" Really Mean?

1. S. B. Roberts, P. Fuss, M. B. Heyman, et al., "Control of Food Intake in Older Men," *Journal of the American Medical Association* 272, no. 20 (1994): 1601–6.

2. U.S. Department of Health and Human Services, "Dietary Guidelines for Americans, 2005." Available at www.health.gov/dietaryguidelines/dga2005/document/pdf/DGA2005.pdf (accessed July 26, 2009).

3. D. Ornish, J. Fletcher, J.-M. Fullsack, and H. R. Roe, *Everyday Cooking with Dr. Dean Ornish: 150 Easy, Low-Fat, High-Flavor Recipes* (New York: HarperCollins, 1996).

4. Q. Sun, M. Jing, C. Hannia, et al., "A Prospective Study of Trans Fatty Acids in Erythrocytes and Risk of Coronary Heart Disease," *Circulation* 115 (2007): 1858–65.

5. M. Schultze, J. Manson, D. Ludwig, et al., "Sugar-Sweetened Beverages, Weight Gain, and Incidence of Type 2 Diabetes in Young and Middle-aged Women," *Journal of the American Medical Association* 292, no. 8 (2004): 927–34.

6. M. G. Tordoff and A. M. Alleva, "Effect of Drinking Soda Sweetened with Aspartame or High-Fructose Corn Syrup on Food Intake and Body Weight," *American Journal of Clinical Nutrition* 51, no. 6 (1990): 963–69.

7. University of Sydney, "The Glycemic Index and GI Database." Available at www.glycemicindex.com (accessed July 26, 2009).

Chapter 3: Dietary Strategies for Hot Flashes, Insomnia, and Other Menopausal Symptoms

1. www.nof.org/professionals/research/nofresearchagenda.

Chapter 4: Understanding Soy Foods: The Perfect Food for Menopause

1. M. M. Seibel, *The Soy Solution for Menopause: The Estrogen Alternative* (New York: Simon & Schuster, 2003).

Chapter 5: More Helpful Foods for Menopause and Other Dietary Guidelines

1. University of Massachusetts Medical School, Center for Integrative Medicine, "Omega-3 Fatty Acids (Fish Oils)." Available at www.umassmed.edu/uploadedfiles/Omega3FattyAcids.pdf (accessed July 20, 2009).

2. T. J. Key, P. N. Appleby, E. A. Spencer, et al., "Cancer Incidence in British Vegetarians," *Cancer* 101 (2009): 192–97.

3. University of Massachusetts Medical School, "Lipids: What Do My Cholesterol Levels Mean?" Available at www.umassmed.edu/healthy heart/tip sheets/lipids.aspx (accessed July 20, 2009).

4. U.S. Department of Agriculture (USDA). "MyPyramid.gov: Steps to a Healthier You." Available at www.mypyramid.gov (accessed July 20, 2009).

5. Centers for Disease Control (CDC)/National Center for Health Statistics (NCHS), National Health and Nutrition Examination Survey (NHANES), NCHS data brief number 17, May 2009. Available at www.cdc.gov/nchs/data/databriefs/db17.htm (accessed August 3, 2009).

6. U.S. Department of Agriculture (USDA), "Inside the Pyramid: What Counts as a Cup of Vegetables?" Available at www.mypyramid.gov/pyramid/vegetables_counts_table.html (accessed July 20, 2009).

7. M. M. Seibel and H. K. Khalsa, *A Woman's Book of Yoga* (New York: Penguin Putnam, 2002).

8. U.S. Department of Agriculture (USDA). "Inside the Pyramid: What Counts as a Cup of Fruit?" Available at www.mypyramid.gov/pyramid/fruits_counts_table.html (accessed July 20, 2009).

9. Centers for Disease Control (CDC), "How to Use Fruits and Vegetables to Help Manage Your Weight." Available at www.cdc.gov/healthyweight/healthy_eating/fruits_vegetables.html (accessed July 20, 2009).

10. University of Massachusetts Medical School, Center for Integrative Nutrition, "Seven Ways to Size Up Your Portions." Available at www.umassmed.edu/uploadedfiles/SevenWaysToSizeUpYour Portions.pdf (accessed July 27, 2009).

11. Siebel and Khalsa.

12. D. Ornish, J. Fletcher, J.-M. Fullsack, and H. R. Roe, *Everyday Cooking with Dr. Dean Ornish* (New York: HarperCollins; 1996).

INDEX